Buh Bye, M.S.

A True Story

Claudia Suzanne

Iridescent Orange Press • Wambtac Communications LLC

This book is not intended for the purpose of providing medical advice. All content of this book is for informational purposes only and is not intended to serve as a substitute for the consultation, diagnosis, and/or medical treatment of a qualified physician or healthcare provider. The reader should regularly consult a physician in matters relating to his/her health and particularly with respect to any symptoms that may require diagnosis or medical attention.

To the fullest extent permitted by law, Claudia Suzanne, Wambtac Communications LLC, and all of their affilates make no representation or warranty as to the reliability, accuracy, usefullness, adequacy or suitability of the information contained in this book.

Although the author and publisher have made every effort to ensure that the information in this book was correct at press time, the author and publisher do not assume and hereby disclaim any liability to any party for any loss, damage, or disruption caused by errors or omissions, whether such errors or omissions result from negligence, accident, or any other cause.

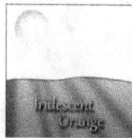

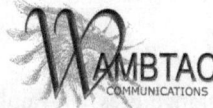

Santa Ana, California

Now and evermore, for Tom

CONTENTS

CONTENTS

DECLARATION

I got rid of multiple sclerosis.

I didn't just beat it or overcome its grip on my life. It's not simply in remission. The scoundrel is absent from my body for the first time in at least 42 years.

Buh bye, M.S.!

Some people find this remarkable. Hey—me, too! And wonderful. And life-affirming. And all those other fantastic adjectives people spout when an incredibly good thing happens to counterbalance all the ugh and icky of the world.

"How did you do it?" people ask. I'll do my best to explain.

Please note: I do not recommend or advocate anything. My victory wasn't fast, easy, or one-size-fits-all. This is simply the story of how I got rid of a cretin that had squatted, uninvited and unwelcome, in my corporeal mass—not how you can get rid of yours. My life has always been complex; the M.S. was merely one more complication that kept trying to take center stage. I had to knock out a bunch of spotlights and install a trapdoor to keep it at bay, but now it's gone, gone, gone. Permanently. Irrevocably. Absolutely.

Does it sound like I considered M.S. a sentient foreign invader?

Yeah, I did.

ONE MORE PROVISO...

Much of my life died with my husband. He had the memory; I had the analysis. That's part of how we divided up life. The other parts are none of your beeswax.

Remember that old joke: "What's the matter with you? Did someone drop you on your head when you were a baby?"

That was me. Not purposely, of course. And I wasn't so much 'dropped' as I managed to fall down the stairs and stop myself on an iron radiator—forehead first. Only a few stitches because mine was a small head. Before that, I'd been a speedy, adroit little thing, on my feet and pushing furniture around at six months. Afterwards, I could trip over changes in a carpet pattern. No one made the connection for about, oh, fifty-two, fifty-three years. By then, I'd given myself two more concussions: one by ducking under an iron bar to get onstage and one by falling face first on the concrete sidewalk when a turbulent patch of air sprang up about half-an-inch off the ground and tripped me.

Ergo, I have a few memory problems.

Of course, my M.S. contributed a few more wrinkles to my total un-recall, but I can't pretend it caused all my long/short-term memory lapses. I distinctly remember—I know; ironic, huh?—the first time I realized that I couldn't remember what I'd known just a few minutes earlier.

Fifth-grade French. I'd studied all night for the conversational exchange and had understood through the entire first row's recital. He said, "Blah blah blah"; she responded, "Blah blahdedity blah." All in perfect French. My row's turn. Got up there in front of the class with my randomly chosen partner. I said, "Blah blah blah"; he responded, "Blah blahdedity blah." My accent was lousy, but my words were perfect. Walked back to my desk. Next couple, same words.

I couldn't understand what they were saying.

No, it wasn't temporary. It wasn't thank-goodness-that's-over relief. It was gone. Gone, gone, gone. I opened my book and looked at the words: they were foreign to me, and I don't just mean because they were in French. All the meaning, even the pronunciation was forgotten. Never came back.

But I remember the incident!

A few years ago, I discovered this kind of memory lapse is called Intermittent Amnesia, and it comes from being hit in the noggin too many times in the exact places I kept introducing my skull to blunt objects.

It only took me decades to remember to write it down so I could remember to look it up.

But none of that has anything to do with my M.S., other than when I was first diagnosed and my husband had to fill out a bunch of forms for...whatever the reason was...he kept writing, "Memory problems getting noticeably worse." When we handed the forms to—well, it probably doesn't matter who, but I remember it was a she and she had a slightly chubby face— she asked, "What do you mean by '...getting noticably worse?'" Tom turned to me and asked a question I don't remember and probably didn't have the answer to then, either, and she looked at me strangely, and he rolled his eyes, and yeah, I remember all *that* but NOT what the question was or what my answer wasn't.

This recitation of how I expelled multiple sclerosis from my body may be spotty in places because so is my memory. Not all the time. But enough that when anyone brings it up in my house, all my kids do the eye-roll thing.

I have four kids. Gave birth to one. Didn't adopt any. Long story for another time, but we all live together and they watched me evict M.S. during the tail-end of its infestation of my chassis. They would all attest to my memory problems if I remembered to ask them, but to what end? The eye rolling gets old.

Oh! One absolutely final word before I actually start getting to the point: if anyone remembers anything differently from the way I put it forth herein, please feel free to write your corrections and comments.

In your own damn book.

For the record, a lousy memory is a boon for a ghostwriter. I never have to worry about maintaining my clients' confidentiality because chances are I won't remember any of the details six months after we finish it. This is called putting a positive spin on things, and it's what I do for a living—so don't go rolling your eyes about that, either!

SET THE SCENE

I have no recollection of my life as a toddler. I don't remember pushing around the furniture, falling down the stairs, or turning into a klutz. That's all hearsay, although I can still see the scar mixed in with the wrinkles on my forehead. Ergo, I am always a bit envious when clients can recite in perfect detail events that occurred at ages two and three. Here's what I do remember.

I grew up in Skokie, Illinois, where some of my neighbors had numbers tattooed on their arms and the Nazis marched to renew the pain long after I left.

My first best friend was Andy. He lived across the street, and we played in the snow with spoons. We married when we were five. When I later found out the marriage wasn't legal, I figured it was just as well since I didn't like his room as much as mine. I had a lot more books. We never played out in the snow for long, though, because I always got cold quickly and deeply and wanted to go back inside. I didn't play in the heat too long, either, because I burned easily, which gave me the *schroshkies*. Not spelled right. Figure it out.

I liked sleeping. I wasn't one of those kids who had to be forced to go to bed. More often, I was watching the clock, waiting for the time I could go up to my room without exasperating my parents. Not that I fell asleep easily. I lay awake for a good hour or more, thinking, goofy-gaming (a.k.a. daydreaming), and sometimes astral traveling, which I assumed (and still unreasonably assume) everyone did and does. When I finally did fall asleep, I slept hard and long. I loved to sleep.

I still love to sleep. It's one of my favorite activities.

I enjoyed astral traveling, even though on the male-to-female spectrum I always knew I wasn't quite all the way over on the female side. Plus, I was never comfortable in my own skin. Consequently, looking down at my body from the ceiling was always something of a shock. I didn't look like what I thought I did—and for some reason, I always looked before I took off to other places.

Later, when I would tell someone about the not-comfortable-in-my-skin thing (or the astral travel thing), they would back away from me with "that look."

I've known "that look" my whole life. I would have preferred those two boys in second grade had given "that look" instead of catching my legs up in a long jump rope and dragging me across the black top while teachers all over the field ignored my scream-ing. Back in class, my teacher Miss Cheney, who was never in a bad mood, was in a bad mood that day and became exasperated when she heard me crying at the rear row.

"What's the matter with you now?" she demanded.

I was too busy crying to answer so the boy next to me said, "Well, she is awfully bloody."

The next day when the two boys apologized, the incident was expunged from the record. After all, boys will be boys. My mother was angry, but my father never even mentioned it—I wasn't even sure he or my brother knew it happened. Years later when I met my future husband, Tom, I still could not talk about it without crying. He got furious—*furious*—and demanded the boys' names. I didn't give them to him, but I never cried over it again.

Sometimes when I lay in bed, my right hand felt like a roll of toilet paper with a wire running across it. My mother told me I had a vivid imagination. What I actually had was later diagnosed as Thoracic Outlet Syndrome (TOS), but such a thing did not exist in medical annals at that time. Now we know it's caused by a cervical rib, a congenital anomaly that rests on the neurovascular bundle in my upper right chest. I am right-handed, so TOS is the reason I couldn't throw the ball, catch the ball, or hold my flute up at the proper angle. At the time, however, "you're just being lazy" was the accepted explanation.

I never wanted to play flute in the first place, but Mom said a clarinet or oboe was not appropriate for a girl. Besides, the reed would only accentuate my buck teeth. Still, I wasn't bad at the flute. I landed second chair every year behind first-chair Donna, who was superb and could play the piccolo.

"You'd be a better flute player if you'd just stop being so lazy and hold your arm up properly," my music teacher/conductor always chided. I tried, but within a few instants the darn thing would droop back down. Obviously, I was too lazy to stop myself from being lazy.

I was also too lazy to run. I was too lazy to ride my bike for more than a few blocks without stopping to rest. Now we know I had—well, have—MVP, Mitral Valve Prolapse (my life is filled with acronyms, isn't yours?), which sapped my stamina. *Then*, the fact that I would not push myself enough to get my heart rate down was undeniable sloth. Fortunately, I was a girl, and a not all-that-bright girl, so what did it really matter?

Okay, I wasn't dumb, I just wasn't fast. My brother, father, and father's relatives were all fast talking, fast thinking, and brilliant. Their IQs were way up the scale. If my genius brother ever brought home something less than an A, it had to be in what we used to call "gym" and is now referred to as P.E., or physical education. Remember, this was the era when only results, not effort, mattered and he couldn't really run either. But he had asthma—a good, legitimate excuse—so all was well. In everything else, he got all As.

On those rare occasions when I got an A, I could count on at least one family member saying: "See? I knew you could do better if you tried."

So my brother, with his photographic memory, read the book once and got As; I studied my butt off and got Bs and Cs. But as long as I did my best, that's all anyone could really ask of me. After all, I was a girl. What did it really matter?

Buh Bye, MS.

Somewhere deep inside, my psyche saw a pattern in all this, but that, too, is for another time. We're here to talk about multiple sclerosis.

When big brother Richard got mono and hepatitis at age nine, I got mono, too. He was two and a half years older than me, the ideal spacing, and never had to play with me (yeah, that's the way Mom put it; don't go there) because our next-door neighbor, who had three boys, told my mother he shouldn't have to. Thus, we were raised completely separately, so it's a wonder that when he got mono, I did, too.

I didn't have asthma or hepatitis, but the doctor told me emphatically that, "Six is too young to have mono." Since I *was* six and I *had* mono, I'd obviously done something horribly wrong. This was more than laziness, this was outright malfeasance.

Bad Claudia! Getting mono at six years old! What were you thinking? Go to your room right now, young lady, and be sick!

And so I was. From that point on, my glands swelled up every time I got a cold or the flu. Swollen glands meant exhaustion, a bad headache, blurry vision, and up to a week (or two) in bed, reading, coloring, dozing, astral traveling, and taking pills. I was sick so often during elementary school I probably swallowed a pharmaceutical shelf of antibiotics. Could all this have added to my lack of stamina and inability to retain test material?

Nah! I was just being lazy. Not lazy myself, you understand, just *being* lazy.

What a shame. And I was such a pretty girl. Why couldn't I learn to apply myself?

I don't remember how old I was when I stepped on the three rusty nails. They were sticking up from a single board and went right through my Keds into the middle of my foot (don't remember which one). I screamed.

(I screamed when I came into my room and found a mouse jumping up and down in my wastepaper basket, too. I had a healthy scream.)

A girl who lived across the street from the empty lot we were playing in yelled that her mother was a nurse and ran to get her. This empty corner lot later sprouted a house where we built a homecoming float—*the* homecoming float, the one Mrs. Todd said caused my extended illness and hospitalization in my sophomore year of high school. She was wrong, but I don't hold it against her. What I hold against her is the D on my James Baldwin's *Go Tell it on a Mountain* paper, not to be confused with the trouble I got into over *Cry, The Beloved Country* in freshman Honors English with an entirely different teacher (whose name I thankfully cannot recall) who once wrote on a paper of mine: "Who do you think you are, the Queen of Sheba? No one is interested in your opinion!"

Ah, yes, in those days, educators bent over backwards to nurture and support their students. This was the same teacher who told the smartest kid in our class of about 500 students that his opinion was wrong. A hellova thing to say. It stopped the entire class. Thirty-two pairs of deer-in-the-headlights stares.

Historians who think the sixties were about nothing but sex and drugs might want to peek a bit below the surface now and then.

But I digress.

Don't remember going to the emergency room when I stepped on the nails, but I'm sure we did. Do remember having to wear gym shoes for a couple of weeks and limping a lot. "Too late for ice now, soak it in hot water," became a mantra in my house after repeated trips to the ER.

By the way, that's a crock. Ice always reduces pain and swelling, no matter when the injury. I know. Long before I became a ghostwriting expert, I was an injury expert.

Don't remember how many years later I went into the garage to get my bike so I could ride the short block-and-a-half to Denise Dorn's house.

Denise Dorn's birthday is April 8th. Can someone please tell me why I remember that?! She is no relation, by the way, to Michael Dorn, the actor who played Worf on *Star Trek: The Next Generation*, although Denise's brother's name was Alan Dorn and when I first saw the *TNG* credits it seemed wrong somehow that they weren't related, despite Alan Dorn being a tall, skinny Jew and the Klingon Michael Dorn being a muscular African-American. I mean, how many Dorns are there in the world?

Yes, this really is the way my brain works; having multiple sclerosis did nothing to improve it.

I never got to Denise's house that day because, unbeknownst to me, a piece of wood lay on the floor of the garage right next to my bike. *That* nail went deep into my right heel, so I screamed, jumped onto my left foot to pull the nail out and landed—aw, come on, you've gotta see where this is going, right?—on another board with another nail that went into my other, i.e., left, heel.

My screaming was loud enough that Harold, the neighbor on the far side from the garage, heard me in the back of his house but not so much that my father, sitting in the living room in the front of our house, noticed until Harold brought me to the door in his arms. I'm sure we went to the emergency room at Skokie Valley Hospital.

We always did. I knew the place well.

The thing about being awkward and no one believing you're not just lazy is that you end up absorbing a awful lot of radiation following accidents and/or gym class, wherein teachers insist you can, so you try but—*Omigod, are you okay?*—you actually can't. Doctors didn't worry about stuff like excessive exposure at the time, so I got x-rayed when I couldn't do a handstand in gym and separated my shoulder (right). I got x-rayed when the field-hockey ball, a solid-wood orb the size of a softball, hit and permanently dented my collar bone (left). (The doctor said he'd never seen anything like it. I cannot tell you how much better that made me feel.)

I got x-rayed when the baseball hit me in the eye (right), and when I fell running (what the hell was I doing running?) out to my mother's car and broke my elbow (I'm guessing either right or left). I got x-rayed when the movable parallel bars ran over my feet, plural. (Don't ask; I was standing still but apparently nevertheless managed to be in the wrong place at the wrong time.) All this happened during elementary school, my "growing" years, when I outgrew and out-developed all but one other girl in my grade, and thus attracted the kind of delightful attention from the boys that all the other girls wished they could get and I would have gladly given away.

I was out of sync like that in a lot of ways. Everyone loved David McCallum in *The Man From Uncle*. I liked Robert Vaughn. "Can't you try to be like the other girls?" my mother would ask. As Raymond Chandler would say, there was nowhere to go with that, so I let it pass.

In high school, I was put into remedial P.E.—yeah, that's what it was called, what a way to pump up the 'ol self-esteem, eh?—with a couple of other klutzes. We weren't allowed to go anywhere near the equipment. No trampoline for us! No ropes or parallel bars or rings or horses or whatever the rest of that stuff-I-wasn't-even-allowed-to-touch was called. No one expected us to do pull-ups (earlier attempts were not fun; just back away from that, okay?) or push-ups (oh, please). Not one of us could return a volleyball, tennis ball, or badminton birdie.

On Parents Day, the only two moms that showed up for gym session were mine and Linda's. We were partners in non-coordination, unrelated twins of unrelated motions, interchangeable butterfingered clods. *Why did you swing there? The ball was nowhere near your racket?!* And yet, we were both tall, thin, and pretty—and she was a natural blonde, to boot. So, really, what did it matter?

I flunked tennis five times in the space of three years. This is not an easy thing to do; I had to flunk it twice in summer school to pull it off. *Today*, an ophthalmologist would look at my lack of hand-eye coordination and see a peripheral-vision problem. *Then...* surely, you can fill in the blanks by now, can't you? Lazy. Uncoordinated. Maybe I walked too early. Well, yeah, I did. Maybe that and my adventure around the black top in second grade somehow impacted my spine. So what? None of that would matter if I'd just learn to stand up straight and hold myself with some pride. My mother sent me to modeling school to fix said issues, which were going to hurt my looks if I didn't learn to overcome my gawkiness. Trust me, this did not help. A lot. But I had such a beautiful figure, and I was so pretty...oy.

Let it snow, let it snow, let it snow.

Buh Bye, MS.

It was into this ill-fitting, slightly twisted, immune-deficient corporeal mass that my rotten-to-the-core adversary, multiple sclerosis, snuck in on the stinger-tip of some cowardly, anonymous mosquito in the fall of the most turbulent year in post-WWII American history: 1968.

Boy, what a lousy year that was.

1968

The Tet Offensive, when the communists lost on the ground but won in the media. Martin Luther King: murdered. Seventy-five percent of NYU students admitted they'd tried marijuana, a big *gasp! Omigod!* deal back then. Bobby Kennedy: murdered. The Democratic Convention, when Mayor Richard J. Daley threw up redwood fences along the entire length of the expressway from O'Hare Airport to downtown Chicago so visitors couldn't see the slums they were passing, and then sent the police to batter and arrest war protesters, thus creating the worst disaster conceivable.

J. Edgar Hoover declared war on the Black Panthers while civil rights activists clashed with police, and what would become known as "the silent majority"—a euphemism for "the frightened complacent"—decried integration. Bigotry abounded on all sides. Americans killed each other with increasingly justifiable (*not*) passion.

And I got bitten by a mosquito.

Actually, I got bitten by what felt like a swarm of mosquitoes. Quick background: Skokie is a twenty-minute bus ride from Chicago, just on the other side of Evanston. You could walk to the elevated (El) station if you were in a sprightly mood; you could ride your bike faster than riding the bus because you didn't have to make stops to pick up and let off passengers.

Buh Bye, MS.

This is all hearsay for me. I never walked or rode my bike to the El. I took the bus when I worked in Skokie and lived in Rogers Park, a subsection of Chicago, but not when I was a kid. As a kid, I wasn't allowed to go to the city by myself or with my friends. My brother was. All my friends were. But not me.

As Joe used to say in *Wings,* "Maybe it's for the best."

The point is we were all of maybe thirty minutes away from Lake Michigan, known for the dead alewives that washed up on the shore every summer, the resulting stink, the wind with its own personality and agenda, and hordes of mosquitoes. More than hordes. Battalions. Whatever is bigger than battalions: armies, maybe. Navies. Marines. Lots and lots of mosquitoes that, not satisfied with the meager thousands who packed the lakeshore every day, spread out across the city and into the suburbs. Suburbs like, oh, say, Skokie, where I, in my innocence, wore short shorts and sleeveless tops against the humidity-laden heat.

It rains in the summer in Chicago, thunderstorms with lots of lightning that leave behind little pondettes and puddles.

Mosquitoes love standing water. Someplace to refresh their tired wings. Someplace to wash their tired feet. Someplace from which to zip out, attack, and retreat before anyone can swat them dead.

Mosquitoes loved me almost as much as their stagnant watering holes. I spent most of my Midwestern summers covered with their love bites, the little shits. But that summer, at least one branch of their military had visited a seriously baaaddd stretch of mud somewhere, and by early to mid-Fall, kids with meningitis were piling up in hospitals all over the area.

I didn't have meningitis. Probably. Maybe. Could be. No one knew for sure. What they did know was that my swollen glands, headaches, and blurred vision weren't responding to antibiotics the way they usually did. My blood tests were alarming but inconclusive.

I didn't care about any of that. All I cared about was that I felt lousy. I couldn't get enough sleep, and I slept constantly. I spent more days in bed than in school. One day when I felt up to trudging the hallways, I discovered that the fastest way to get from the top of the Niles East professional auditorium to the bottom two floors down was to simply pass out in mid-step near the top and come around tangled up somewhere just above the floor with your girl-friend screaming in your ear and feeling you over for blood.

No serious blood, no broken bones. When one passes out, one goes totally limp; ergo, the fall, which I admit I don't remember, was loose. My only injuries were some scrapes and bruises, and—oh, yeah, I forgot about this one—another bump on the head. Probably the back of the head that time, but seriously, I don't remember. Don't remember if I had a concussion, either, but that really didn't matter because my doctor, who was actually my mother's doctor, thought my new method of descending a staircase stunk and stuck me in the hospital.

I spent nine days in St. Joseph Hospital, enjoying it not one lit-tle bit. They did an upper GI and a lower GI. They did a spinal tap and took enough blood to start a new person. They x-rayed my head, because I so seriously needed more radiation exposure. They prob-ably did some other stuff, but God bless my Swiss-cheese memory, I have no idea what that might have been.

Some friends came to see me once; I remember the fact of the crowd but not the actual visit. Did my brother come? My father? Don't remember. Sorry, guys; my bad, not yours.

The most interesting part of being hospitalized—besides being so dizzy and tired and blurry-eyed I couldn't even watch TV despite this being the first time in my life I had a television completely to myself and total control over the remote—was the voices. I heard voices.

They were the same voices I'd heard the previous time I'd been hospitalized in the same hospital in the same kind of room but on a different floor when I was a little girl and something was wrong with my digestive tract. See how nicely I put that? I'd love to say "I'm omitting the gory details out of a sense of delicacy," but come on, you know the truth: I don't remember what was wrong with me.

But Denise Dorn's birthday is forever implanted in my brain. Now why is that?

What I do remember is the rice. Plain boiled rice, every meal for a week. Three times a day: plain boiled rice. Want a snack? How about some nice rice? It was supposed to help my gut.

It helped me hate rice.

"Why was a little girl having digestive problems?" I hear you ask. I suspect stress. Quick version: mine was not an...uh...easy household. Nobody put their hands on anybody, nothing like that. Just a lot of...uh...let's use the word *tension*. Guess you've got to understand the people involved in order to understand the dynamics of the situation.

My brother Richard really was a genius. IQ tests proved it, and his damned photographic memory demonstrated it all the time. He wasn't alone. Everyone in Dad's family was irritatingly smart: Aunt Ruth was erratically brilliant, first-cousin David was infuriatingly gifted, and first-cousin Jack was quietly an egghead. They all had logical, methodical, problem-solving minds and personalities.

My mother dreamt of being a singer, ala Judy Garland, or an actress ala Ava Gardner (look it up). Mom had a wonderful voice and a deep-seated love of being center stage, but her parents had inculcated her with the idea that she was stupid, worthless, and a major disappointment in the general scheme of humanity, so—surprise, surprise—her dreams went by the wayside. She spent her entire girlhood longing for the kind of smoldering true love Heathcliff had for Catherine in *Wuthering Heights*, a movie she watched over fifty times instead of going to school. She married my father, she told me numerous times (although I didn't believe her), because he was a nice Jewish boy who adored her and grandma wasn't interested in any more stalling. I'm encapsulating. Extensively. To put it simply, my parents were/are an...interesting match.

They both loved to dance.

The point is Mom was nice; she liked things "pretty." (Please don't ask how I came from her; the universe is full of unfathomable mysteries.) She was also a pretty savvy lady but had learned to not show it—not that it mattered, because raising a genius when you're not one yourself is no easy task. I know of what I speak: Tom's paternal line also leaned way over into gifted and the combination of our genes produced a daughter whose IQ outranks mine by a good twenty, maybe forty points, probably more. She could outthink me by the time she was seven or eight. Fortunately, though, she has my sweet, adorable nature, so all is well.

Hey, my story, my perspective.

Mom may not have been able to outthink Rich, but she knew right from wrong, and it was only right to expect deference from her son due to the simple fact that she was his mother.

Maybe Rich didn't believe in deference, or maybe he was just a normal, gifted kid who couldn't understand why his mom didn't understand him. This is probably a false encapsulation, but whatever. Here's how dinner time went at least two or three times a week at our house:

Rich said something that raised Mom's hackles. Mom called him on it. Rich snapped back at her, voice rising. She bawled him out, he hollered at her, and then—now, here's the tricky part—Dad yelled at Mom, who snapped and shouted some more until everyone was loud enough that Dad slammed the table in fury to end the whole mess.

I sat in the only seat from which one could not easily vacate the scene. A captive audience to this recurring performance, I was hemmed in by Mom to my right, the wall to my left, and the refrigerator directly behind. Everyone else had an exit strategy.

Since I cannot claim accurate recall, neither can I categorically point to stress as the root cause of my stomach problems, but I'd be willing to put real money on it, even up to $2.97 or all the way to $3.46.

Which brings me back to the week-long, plain boiled-rice adventure during which I heard voices. Not, I quickly learned, voices coming from the nurses' desk, the bed next to me, the people in the rooms on either side of me, or the televisions from any of the above. The voices talked on top of each other, and I could never make out what anyone was saying. My mom chalked it up to goofy-gaming. The nurses said I was dreaming. I put my hands over my ears, but when I pulled them away, the voices were there again. Maybe it's coming from the pipes, someone said.

Now, that didn't make any sense. Why would a bunch of people go into a pipe to whisper to each other late at night? And just how big was this pipe, anyway?

But the same voices were there all those years later (however many years that was), doing exactly the same thing, talking on top of each other, whispering in snatches, every night, all night, when I was confined for over a week so the powers-that-be could poke, prod, and medically molest me.

Now that I think of it, they were there some three-and-a-half decades later in another St. Joseph's Hospital, this one in Orange, California, where my husband went to not be treated for Stage 4 cancer, a condition we didn't know he had until one month, exactly, before he died. In the new order of hospitalization, family is now encouraged to stay all night, ostensibly for the patient's comfort but in practice for the patient's needs. Neither of us slept all that well no matter which garret he was assigned at the time, but whenever I took the ear buds out in the quasi-quiet of the deep night, there they were: the same voices. I suspect they were the whispers of past patients held captive in their rooms of medical dread, but it's possible I watch too much *Star Trek* and *Doctor Who*.

In any event, the upshot of all those tests and medication failures after my teenage nine-day confinement was presented to my mother on a visit to the doctor's office after I'd been released from St. Joseph's and had returned—headache, blurry vision, dizziness, bone-weary fatigue, and all—to school.

"Multiple Sclerosis."

No, no, wait! Don't touch that dial, because you just don't know my mother.

The doctor said, "M.S."

My mother said, "No."

And that was it. End of discussion. *Excuse me, Mr. Fancy Pants M.D., but you can take your M.S. and put it where the sun don't shine.*

Being a fifteen-year-old child with no rights whatsoever, I was not, of course, in the room. I don't even know if I was there at all, to be honest. But Mom drove home crying, and by the time she reached the house, those ugly, disgusting initials had been safely locked away in some inaccessible cell cluster in a remote sector of her brain, never to be seen or heard from again.

She told no one. Anything. Ever. Period.

Until 1999. Or was it 2009?

I don't remember.

If Tom was here, he'd know.

The amazing thing is: my not knowing didn't stop the M.S.

Can you believe that?

TOM NINETEEN-NINETY-NINE.

Tom isn't here to tell me, but my daughter remembers we found out about the 1968 diagnosis in 1999, because she had a telemarketing job that summer and came home one day excited about a big sale only to find her father ranting around the house.

"She knew! She fucking knew all along! How the fuck could she not tell us! Jesus fucking Christ, Claudi!"

My apologies for the gutter-language; I just wanted to give you the flavor of his speech pattern. Won't happen again.

Probably.

Perhaps this is a good point to further introduce Tom, since, after all, he was an integral part of how I dealt with, battled, and ultimately vanquished our mutual foe—and also because I met him the year I was diagnosed and lost him the year I recognized the bastard's absence from my body.

Remarkable coincidence, huh?

Yeah, right.

Tom and I met twice that summer before the mosquito strike: once outside Niles East and once at Susie's house. Those were both more encounters than actual meetings, but we nevertheless immediately knew that we knew each other, even though we did not yet know each other. And despite sensing an immediate and irrepressible draw to each other, neither of us wanted to have much to do with the other at the time, except to spend time together.

Please. Don't even ask.

It was some decades before we realized we'd played out this dance before in at least one, if not several, previous incarnations. At that particular point in this particular go-around, however, our appearance in each other's lives was instantaneously irritating, reassuring, sensually (but not sexually) charged, and just altogether too damn comfortable for either of our comfort. During our best times over the next forty-two years, we needed a lot of space from each other. During our worst times, we screamed at each other.

"I LOVE YOU!"

"YEAH? WELL I LOVE YOU, TOO!"

Another interesting match. They run in the family.

Jumping back to the M.S.: since no one acknowledged that I had it, I was never treated for it, and my headache, blurry vision, dizziness, clumsiness, lack of balance, exhaustion, etc. just disappeared some six or seven months after they started. People clued into their diagnosis would recognize this as remission in a remitting/relapsing course of the disease. Since the concept of such an illness never entered my family's consciousness, our take was that I'd either had a miraculous recovery or "whatever it was" had simply run its course. Take your pick. Didn't matter. Life went on.

Here's the kicker, though: when "whatever it was" went away, it didn't take my recurring swollen glands, weariness, blurry vision, clumsiness, etc., *et. al,* with it. They came back now and then, here and there, like Harvey, the pooka. We should have bought stock in the company that made ampicillin; we could have gotten wealthy just from my consumption. But it always worked—or it worked good enough—so what's the point of bellyaching?

This made no sense from any and all angles, but thank God there wasn't anything really wrong with me. I didn't go out much in high school, because I preferred to hit the sack early. And I slept in late so often on the weekends that one of my friends said it was pointless to call me before 10:30 in the morning since I'd either still be in bed or just getting into the shower.

I was tired. Bone-tired. Constantly, constantly weary. And the more I exercised, the more I pushed through, the more I made myself stay up and dance (never made it through a single full tune, never, not once), the more tired I got. I couldn't quite hit any of the notes I was supposed to hit in mixed chorus, either, no matter how much I practiced, because I couldn't seem to figure out the intricacies of breath control. The more I tried, the more it wore me out.

Obviously, I wasn't trying hard enough. Obviously, I was just being lazy.

I did get into the advanced singing class the first semester of my junior year when I somehow found the voice to hit an amazing note—one I've never hit since, by the way, and o! how I would have loved to get that note back when Tom and I were on the road, but no, it was a one-time, one-note performance. Hope you were present for its appearance because we shall never hear of such a note again. I didn't last in choir, though, because, well, a) I never hit that note again, and b) I had to go running out in the middle of class one day due to a Reynaud's attack.

Okay, backing up—did I mention the Reynaud's before? A hereditary vascular condition wherein the capillaries in one's hands and feet go into spasm when one gets too cold. Or too stressed. That day I got too cold, and my protector—a.k.a. Tom, a.k.a. someone else's boyfriend, and just what the hell was he doing hanging around with someone like me?—explained to our director and his mentor, Mr. Auge, that I couldn't handle the air conditioning. (The choir room was the only one in the entire school not hot and humid during summer and frosted over in the winter.)

Auge didn't find Tom's explanation plausible or amusing.

As soon as school let out that year, my family moved from Skokie, Illinois to Orange, California because my mother's Reynaud's was not going to make it through another winter without her either driving her 1965 Dodge convertible off a cliff or destroying her liver with the then-accepted medication-of-choice for Reynaud's: brandy.

These were gentler times; she had a prescription to carry an open bottle in her car.

I was thrilled to leave Skokie, the world's biggest village, so named because the local pols refused to upgrade it to a town. I was essentially a nonentity in school until I wrote a couple of articles that bit me in the ass—then and, amazingly, decades later, when Tom's high-school ex and her husband came to see him play and she asked me, "Did you really mean it when you wrote that story for the school newspaper claiming you were a witch, or were you just fucking with everybody?"

Actually, I seem to recall I was a member of a coven at the time, but I told her it was a little bit of both, because, frankly, I didn't remember my motivation for writing the article. Besides, my brain could not wrap itself around the idea that someone would actually remember a throw-away article in a high-school newspaper thirty-eight years earlier. So I elaborated, as is my wont (or hadn't you noticed?) by pointing out that Miriam, Moses' sister, was Wiccan, a claim that may or may not be true, but which I picked up who-knows-where and sure sounded good at the time. It startled the ex enough that her eyes went wide.

But I digress.

I was also glad to leave the Midwest because I hated the cold, I got sick and bitten up every summer (no M.S. clues there, nosiree!), and the only people I was likely to miss were my friends Liz and Jackie. For some inexplicable reason, I didn't think about missing Tom because if I had, I would have just shrugged, knowing he'd always be there.

I knew that because...? Not a clue.

Tom loved telling the story of how he walked over to my vacated house the day after we left and mused, "How can I marry her if she's moved to California?"

We had never dated. We never did, in fact. I don't know why. Probably because it was psychically unnecessary. We were so damn connected we spent the next nine years trying to *not* get married. Our mutual efforts didn't work, which is why he was the one who

Buh Bye, MS.

discovered the connection between multiple sclerosis and Evening
Primrose Oil. But that was decades later.

NOT THYROID

By the time my senior class graduated back in Skokie, I had been in and out of the Air Force for three weeks and two days, which was as much as the military and I could take of each other. I didn't mention having Reynaud's on my application medical form and since nothing else was wrong with me, I didn't mention that, either.

Our new California doctor said my mother was a nervous woman and that I was just like her, nervous. That's why I was so tired all the time. Living with her, he said, would make anyone nervous. I needed to get away from the stress of my family. So I moved back to the north side of Chicago and got my own apartment in Roger's Park, but being away from my stressful family didn't make me any less tired. I one time thought my head was going to explode from the pressure and pain of having nothing wrong with me, so I called on my former Chicago doctor, who told me I was getting upset over nothing: it was just the same old/same old headache, exhaustion, clumsiness, and swollen glands I always had.

"Good to see you again, by the way. How's your mom?"

If he knew or even thought I had M.S., he didn't mention it, but then again he also wouldn't let me see my medical records because I was still under twenty-one. Legally, he said, he couldn't show them to me.

Buh Bye, MS.

Sound like a crock to you? Sounded like one to me, too, but in distant retrospect, I suspect he was merely protecting his rear echelon.

No one ever gave any mind to my inability to hang onto things, my consistent failure to clear doorways without scraping one side or the other, my tendency toward non-viral/non-bacterial laryngitis, or the lack of feeling in my feet to the extent that the only way I knew I'd cut myself was when someone noticed the blood trail. All these little peccadilloes were just part of my natural, loveable clumsiness.

I returned to California after breaking up with the lying piece of scum I'd followed back to my hometown (and over whom I lost my best friend) and got an apartment at Wilshire and Berendo in Los Angeles. I earned my keep doing office temp work and salved my soul volunteering evenings at Cedars of Lebanon Hospital, where I saw Tony Fransiosca visit his wife in the maternity ward and cried when Bobby Darin died in the other wing. I decided I wanted to go into the medical profession—but still didn't want to go to college, which is why I had joined the Air Force in the first place; yeah, the logic in those two concepts eludes me at this point, too—so I signed up to become a Licensed Vocational Nurse through a now-defunct program at the now-defunct Queen of Angels Hospital.

Sure, it was a lot for someone with as little stamina as I had, but I didn't want to be lazy. Lots of people work full time while going to school—which is exactly what I said to the doctor in the employee emergency room at Cedars of Lebanon Hospital when I came around after passing out, apparently, at my desk in the admitting office. Couldn't name the current president (Nixon) much less the vice president (Agnew; just showing off that I know the right answers now). Wasn't sure what day of the week it was. Why? Wasn't I scheduled to work that day?

The diagnosis that time was simple exhaustion, brought on by not recognizing that I was *not* one of those people who can work and go to school at the same time. I tossed a coin, my mother caught it, and I started hitting the freeway at 4:30 every morning to get from my parents' house in Orange County up to Los Angeles in time to pick up two classmates and make it to the floor of Queen of Angels by 6:00 AM change-of-shift.

I slept all weekend. All weekend. Every minute of the weekend.

"Don't you ever date?" someone asked.

"There's a guy in Chicago I'm going to marry," I answered, even though we hadn't talked or written at that point for months and neither of us had ever even broached the subject of matrimony. To be honest, it shocked me when I said it, but only because in that instant I knew it was true.

Nursing school didn't work out for me (and I apologize now, publicly, to that teacher I inadvertently got fired. I'd have apologized personally years ago if I could remember her name, face, or nationality. Mine is an equal-opportunity memory lapse), so I took advantage of my Honors at Entrance acceptance to Cal State Fullerton, not yet a university, and started their pre-med program.

All went well the first semester, which was actually the year's second semester, because I didn't have to peer through a microscope, and the guy who joined me on our "on your honor" eighteen-hole golf final didn't feel like doing all eighteen holes, either. We did about five or six and made up the rest on our scorecards, he with an eye to getting me drunk and into bed, me with an eye to just getting into bed, the better to get some sleep. I went along with his version of hitting the sack so I could get to the good stuff, but the next day I didn't feel right, so off to Doctor Jerko I went.

You notice I'm not printing his name. He's still around, currently the head of some hospital and probably as incompetent as ever. I saw him one Christmas season a lifetime or two after I'd disengaged from his medical practice. Recognizing me, he gleefully asked about my husband.

Everyone always asked about Tom first; even teachers he never took classes from knew him. I once went up to a teacher I'd had in elementary school to say hello. She didn't remember me, but that was probably because I was, as one high-school instructor told me, "eminently forgettable," which paired nicely with one my aunts saying, "It's so easy to forget you're around."

Buh Bye, MS.

And the hits just keep on coming.

After assuring Doctor NeverMindHisName that Tom was fine, thank you, I said bluntly, "I have multiple sclerosis"— because by then I knew the truth. The look on his face told me he knew, too. He'd known forever. Why he never wanted me to know back when I haunted his office for answers to my exhaustion and clumsiness is beyond the workings of my simple brain.

Dumbass doctor.

But I didn't know any of this the morning I left my golf partner's bed feeling not very well and went to Doctor MayHisBallsShrive-lUpAndFallOff's office to get checked out. I was so exhausted I fell asleep on the exam table waiting for APoxOnHisNameForever to come in. When he did, he was purely exasperated at having to wake me and told me, without pausing to do an examination or glance at the chart, that there was nothing wrong with me, there had never been anything wrong with me, and I should stop coming to his office and wasting his time.

And that's not the amazing part.

The amazing part is that after Tom and I got married, we actually used MedicalBastardIncorporated as our primary physician, because he was the only physician I knew. Besides, Tom liked him— until the day that he, Tom, witnessed him, Dr. BlowItOutYourButt, talking to me.

I am so glad I never gave in to my husband's demand that we get a gun in the house. He was my protector from start to finish.

Buh bye, Doctor RhymesWithBrick.

But I'm jumping ahead, because Tom and I didn't get married until we already hadn't gotten married four times, and my mother hadn't gotten her deposit back on that Italian-lace dress. But, what the heck, I'll jump ahead because it all boils down to the same dreary refrain—the one every person with multiple sclerosis knows too well: there was nothing wrong with me. The headaches were meaningless, the blurry vision and numbness were my imagination, and what I called "extreme weariness" could be eradicated by a little exercise and better sleep. Did I snore?

I do now, but no, I didn't then. I slept like a log. Whenever I could find someplace horizontal.

It wasn't until we'd been married for a few months (in a judge's chambers, because my mother was not going to plan another wedding, damn it, and Tom felt compelled to stop the car on the outer drive to call her from an emergency phone to tell her that, yes, we were finally, formally, and in all other ways married) that I sustained the permanent back injury driving for 24 Hour Airport Express, another now-defunct operation, that sent me to Dr. Adam Daniels, Chiropractor extraordinaire, who diagnosed all my problems in one swell foop.

Thyroid.

He said my problems were all due to low thyroid output. Or was it high thyroid? Don't remember, doesn't matter, because no, it wasn't thyroid. But he was so sure it was, and we were so glad to have a definitive answer that we bellied up to the bar and laid down our fifty-cent piece.

"Why doesn't it show up on her blood tests?" Tom demanded. Because...well, Adam didn't have an answer to that, but it was obviously thyroid, it had to be thyroid, so we all accepted it was thyroid. No drug pusher, Adam recommended I get a supplement called simply "T," and assured me that if I took it regularly, my exhaustion, headaches, etc., etc., etc. would all disappear over the next six months.

Unfortunately, he was dead before those six months were over, probably from cancer, or perhaps from the stress of having both his wife and pregnant mistress working together in the same office. But he was a great guy. Before he died, he showed Tom how to put my back in (Tom had great hands) and me how to put Tom's back in (not so great, but crudely effective) so that when we went on the road, we could take care of each other.

So we went on the road.

ON THE ROAD

Tom and I decided to hit the road as a husband-wife piano-drums duo because we'd played as many Moose and Elk lodges and military officer and enlisted clubs as we could stand, and because my brother's dog (who lived with my parents but was attached to my husband) and my maternal grandfather both died.

Yes it was impulsive, and yes it was reckless, and yes Tom was a conservative, take-no-chances kinda guy, but one of the things he loved about me was that I brought an element of terrifying excitement into his life. So within a few weeks of Grandpa's funeral, we packed everything into a storage shed—including the Corel cookware we both loved that was mysteriously M.I.A. when we unpacked the shed—and set off to see the country in our 1976 Chevy half-ton van. We were young, we were beautiful, we were as stupid as they come, and if I didn't bring up Tom's pot smoking, he didn't bring up my weary clumsiness or inability to stay on key.

A match made in heaven.

Here's where things get tricky, because although I remember most of the places we played, I don't really remember the order. I'm pretty sure the first gig was Moses Lake, Washington, where the stage sat directly right in front of a single-pane window separating us from the lake. Moses Lake is cold during the middle of winter.

Reynaud's-attack-inducing cold.

The second night we were there, a man casually walked up to the enormous painting at the top of the stairs, stage left, plucked it from the wall, and set it off to the side where apparently no one would notice. Damn me, I noticed, and the waitress, after just as casually returning the painting to its proper position, comp'd me a hot-buttered rum in gratitude.

Enough of those, and my fingers and toes felt warm and toasty, thank you so very much. Welcome to the wonderful world of the traveling musician. Pedal-to-the-metal drives after last call Sunday night/Monday morning so we could be onstage two states away for Tuesday's downbeat. Lots of coffee on the road, lots of booze on the gig, lots of jokes onstage while Tom figured out what tune we were going to do next—and no memory at the end of the night, damn it, of what I'd said to make them laugh so I could hone it for the next show.

Frustrating.

Afternoons, we hunted for vitamin stores—this was before the health-food craze or personal computers—trying to find that "T" Dr. Daniels wanted me to take or at least a reasonable substitute. It wasn't actually helping, but we were sure that in time it would. Meanwhile, we ate like idiots: deep-fried ham sandwiches, a.k.a. Monte Cristos; house-specialty chocolate mousse; and prime rib drenched in sautéed mushrooms and onions every night (when it was on the house). We drank all night and bickered over my inability to stay on pitch and his inability to create a set list all day. My talent was nowhere near the level of Tom's, but my time was usually dead-on. Even so, we rushed through some songs so fast we finished almost before we started. He took no consolation in the fact that the Commodores rushed every tune on their hit albums. I took no consolation in the fact that I could sing harmony against almost anything.

I was better at harmony because for some reason I naturally gravitated to the counter note instead of the melody. I couldn't really sing worth a damn anyway, but my voice against his usually worked. Ever hear "Misty" or "New York, New York" in full harmony, first note to last? It's an experience, one that so enraged a drunk in some bar out in the wilds of somewhere that he kept feeding our tip jar so we'd do it again just to prove we couldn't, nobody could, you can't do that to that kind of song. We were unique and living the good life with "Just the Two of Us" (a ballad we did, by the way, endlessly). We were free, we were healthy, we were in love…

Okay, he was healthy. My body kept slowing down. The more I practiced the worse I got, so I gave up practicing and once we'd nailed down the vocals, we gave up rehearsing, too. If I sounded good at the beginning of the night, I was off-key and dragging the beat by the end. Totally backwards: musicians—all musicians—get better as the evening goes on because they get warmed up and further into the music.

It's a rule, like scientists don't make money and writers aren't meant to understand tech.

I got cold instead of warm, disoriented instead of into it, and exhausted and broken by the time we hit "Pink Panther," our nightly closing tune. Tom needed to run or smoke or find another place to play when we got off stage. I needed bed. I took off my makeup the next morning in the shower. I was lucky to get out of my clothes before I dropped into bed. My hands hurt, my arms ached, my legs stumbled, the top of my head felt like someone was whapping me with a two-by-four.

Next morning, I was fine. We pushed on.

I don't remember where we were after Moses Lake—Edmonton, Alberta, I think—but at some point we got to Terrace, British Columbia, one of the most beautiful spots on earth. Tom made some local-musician friends (read: dealers) right away, so when I didn't duck down far enough to get under that iron bar getting back on stage one night, the drummer took over on for me when we got back from the hospital.

Yes, you read that right. I split my head open, went to the local Canadian fix-it clinic, got patched up—"She probably has a concussion; don't let her fall asleep for the next, 10, maybe 12 hours, eh?

And if the wound keeps oozing, come back tomorrow"—and then went back onstage. What a trooper, huh?

I'm pretty sure I changed my clothes first, since split heads tend to bleed a lot. Don't remember, but I do recall singing "Rolling on the River," or at least some words and notes to that effect, from stage left while Tom's Canadian buddy put me to shame on my own chrome-wrapped Yamaha power drum kit.

Afterwards, my darling hubby put me to bed and then took off with the drummer to enjoy a few tokes at the guy's honest-to-God log cabin, where he stashed his stash between the logs to hide it from the Mounties. He hoisted the wall to snatch the stuff out after his semi-domesticated wolves had sufficiently obfuscated the odor so the pot-detecting German Shepherds couldn't decide where it was. These guys took their arrest avoidance seriously.

I, on the other hand, lay there weirdly awake, trying to get away from the strange sensation in my back that I couldn't stop no matter what position I rolled to. My muscles clenched. Then they ziggled. Clench, ziggle. Clench, ziggle, ziggle, clench. Ziggle, ziggle, clench-clench-clench, ziggle, ziggle, ziggle.

It's called stasis and it's a textbook symptom of M.S., but we didn't have that textbook or even an inkling of that diagnosis. The next day it was gone. Musta come from hitting my head. Or maybe my Reynaud's. I blamed a lot of stuff on Reynaud's. It was a very convenient, and mostly silent, scapegoat.

We went on with our pooka imitation, appearing here and there, now and then, in this place and that, occasionally going home to recoup and then heading out again. At some point, we played the Hyatt or Hilton or Holiday Inn in Rock Springs, Wyoming. The bar was directly behind the stage, separated by a bunch of vertical slats through which, if you were drunk enough, you could grab my ass, and I, in turn, could shove a drum stick up your nose if you touched me one more time, buster.

It was only a threat. I never actually did it. Gimme a break.

One night between sets, we looked in on the very loud "casino extravaganza" in the banquet room at the end of the hall around the corner. Turned out it was a members-only event thrown by the local synagogue—"the" synagogue in the region, as a matter of fact—to raise funds for a new synagogue, a classic Jewish ritual. As soon as the temple president realized we were *lonsmen* (fellow Jews), he invited us to the community's Passover Seder, out of which we had to duck right after permanently clearing our sinuses with the hottest horseradish-on-matzo ever served anywhere, anytime. I can still open my nose just thinking about it.

We were also invited to attend another temple member's bris from hell on Easter Sunday.

It started early in the day, leaving us plenty of time to return to the hotel and nap before work. At least that was the plan.

One more great plan that just didn't work out.

See, the baby cried. The mother tittered around making sure everyone enjoyed the buffet, because, hey, we're Jews, food comes first. Even in Rock Springs, Wyoming, you shouldn't leave without first having a nice piece smoked fish, *nu*? The father strutted with his wailing son, his face scrunching now and then into perfect despair. The *mohel* (a non-rabbi who performs circumcisions) was late, making the big topic of discussion a five-year-old whose face was done up like a model's. This was long before six-year-old Jon Benét got killed and the world discovered no little girl is too young to be made into a sex object. In our crowd of upscale/down home Rock Springs Jews, this little one wisely stuck close to her mother while other moms shook their heads, dads cast sideway glances, and Tom and I stayed within clutch distance of each other. I milled about. He drank. What a great afternoon. Is it time to go yet?

Finally, the mohel arrived and the ceremony began. In a nutshell:

The kid screamed. The father blanched. The grandmother gagged. The baby screeched. The mother cried. The grandfather had to lie down. And then the mohel asked for a sharper knife.

I kid you not.

Two and a half hours later, Tom and I were back at the hotel making our own baby, that very day, Easter Sunday, in Rock Springs,

Wyoming, repeatedly and frantically, trying to block out the scene we'd just witnessed from our minds. It didn't work, but by the time we got onstage, I knew with absolute certainty that I was pregnant.

We both prayed it would be a girl.

And I felt fantastic.

OFF THE ROAD

I had a picture-perfect pregnancy and an equally perfect delivery, playing the drums all the way through my seventh month so my daughter would come out of the womb always able to find one in any tune (as in *one*-two-three-four). I quizzed her on it when she was five. Yup, her rhythm was dead-on.

I had not a single health problem from beginning to end of that pregnancy: no Reynaud's attacks, no that-which-was-not-named, no thoracic this or that. My OB/GYN mentioned a few times that my heart rate was kind of high, but none of us paid it any mind. For nine months, I glowed.

On December 14, 1982, the doc said I'd probably deliver shortly after the first of the year. I said, "No"—hey, like mother, like daughter—and Tom and I set off to walk the baby out. We walked one mall for four hours that day and two malls the next day for eight hours. By 10 PM that second night I had labor twinges. Somewhere around midnight, we called our support person, now Dr. Bera Dordoni, my naturopath, and told her to meet us at the hospital.

We checked into the Santa Ana Western Medical Center's birthing room around 2:30 AM. Ilona Nicholle made her debut later that morning, around 10:30 on Saturday, December 16, 1982, too late for us to perform at the Christmas show we were booked to play at the same hospital that afternoon. Bera subbed for us.

I just this moment realized that my daughter's father died at approximately the same time twenty-seven and a half years later. I only mention it because it's the kind of numerical connection that would have fascinated my mother-in-law, *alev ha sholem.* Tom would have liked it, too. I find I channel him sometimes. Also, it's kinda interesting, especially when you consider that his mother also died about 10:30, also on a Saturday, the day after my birthday. I asked her not to die on my birthday, and she said, "Okay."

In any event, six weeks after Lona was born, the three of us packed our stuff into The Van and its new pull-along equipment trailer and headed for our first post-partum gig in Moberly, Missouri.

Six weeks! I took that precious baby away from her grandmother, my mother, at only six weeks?! What was the matter with me?

Simple: we made our living playing music on the road. Giving birth had taken the last of our nickels, and we had to replenish our bank account or we'd either a) have to continue camping at my parents' house or b) go get real jobs. Neither option made any sense in our young, stupid heads, so we strapped our newborn into a car seat, backwards as per instructions, and headed off in the middle of winter across the Rocky Mountains, through Denver, Colorado, where my brother lived with his girlfriend.

And her boa constrictor.

Which raised its head and stared at me as I sat on the bed and nursed my daughter for, oh, a good half nanosecond before awkwardly but swiftly removing myself, my still-suckling infant, and the requisite bag of baby paraphernalia from the room and informing my husband that no, we weren't going to crash there for the night.

I realize now as I did then that leaving SoCal was not the most popular decision we could have made. Looking back, though, I'm so grateful for those six months the three of us spent just with each other. I don't want to get all gooey, but it was a magical, if sometimes terrifying interlude. And my pregnancy healthiness just kept on going.

Buh Bye, MS.

It all ended some six months later, when Daddy could no longer deal with leaving his daughter in the hands of a new babysitter every time we hit a new town. We had to call on my aunt Shirley to pinch-hit one night after we found our room cluttered with one-too-many used condoms.

Another night we discovered The Van's door standing open when we were dragging out equipment off stage. Nothing was stolen, a good fortune we attributed to Rabbit, our Gund® bunny, and Bear, our Gund®, uh, bear, having frightened the perpetrators off from their position strapped into passenger seat. But that was the last straw for Tom. We borrowed $200 from my aunt Ruth and crossed the country for the last time.

We landed back in SoCal just in time to take a July 4th gig someplace across from Disneyland, so we could oooh and aahh at the fireworks every 9:30 PM for the next however-many-weeks-it-was until we were replaced. The nights were chilly but I was still breast-feeding, so I wrapped myself in useless shawls and moved around a lot. I wasn't playing the drums anymore at this point, which turned out to be both a major mistake and an even bigger advantage.

We went back to doing our pooka imitation but with a few wrinkles: now and then I took a temp typing gig; once, Tom settled himself into a full-time legit job. None of these devices took hold. He was a musician's musician, and I had already put in my office-worker time. Things between us, rocky from the start, got tense and cranky. Pretty soon, we were confronted with that ultimate choice all couples face sooner or later.

The marriage or the act.

A no-brainer, eh? He got a piano gig, feeling nothing but relief. I answered auditions for other groups feeling…lots of other, not-quite-so-wonderful emotions. But neither of us was going to give up our careers or each other, much as we often wanted to. We could hate and spit at each other, but we couldn't leave.

We were joined at the zero-point field.

My first solo audition was *Fucking A!*, musician lingo for everybody had a great time. It was an all-guy band, we jammed for a couple of hours, I was hot! At the end, the leader said, "Yeah, that was good; thanks for coming—but my mom says I can't hire a girl. Sorry." As I loaded my drums into the back of the car, I must have hit my head on the hatchback, because by the time I got home I had a horrific headache, the type that put me down, that made me so dizzy I couldn't see. I hadn't had one like it since...well, I couldn't remember but it had been years, absolutely years. Definitely before the baby. Maybe even before we went on the road; then again, maybe not. I couldn't remember. I didn't care. Horrible headache.

Tom took me to the emergency room—we didn't have a doctor anymore—but they couldn't find any evidence of injury. They sent me home with some naproxen samples and a discharge sheet that said, "Probable M.S."

What?!

No.

I went to another audition the next day, fully expecting to land this one since it was an all-girl band. Apparently, however, sometime during the night some non-musician had snuck into my room and replaced my arms and legs with their own pathetic limbs, because not only couldn't I keep the beat, I couldn't start the beat. I had no strength, no coordination, no syncopation whatsoever. I didn't even have a tail to droop between my legs as I dragged my sorry butt home.

I didn't get the gig.

But I knew I could play! Maybe no one wanted to hear me sing (trust me, no one wanted to hear me sing), but I had recordings and applause and compliments that proved I could play!

Obviously, I was just out of shape from laying off for so long.

Obviously, I just needed to pump myself back into my former lean, mean, drumming machine condition.

So I went to my mother's house to do laps in her pool. Sixty laps up and back, to be exact; that's what I aimed for, that's what I did. I don't know why I picked that number. Not a little pool, either, a good-sized one, shallow on the north end and deep enough on the south to warrant a diving board. I was only thirty, maybe thirty-one years old. I could do this! I'd whip myself back into shape in no time.

The next morning, my right hand would not grasp my daughter's hair brush. It looked like I was wearing a catcher's mitt. Tom freaked. I freaked. The woman at the UCLA Vascular Surgery department freaked and juggled schedules to get us in ASAP. We drove up there angry as bears to find out what the heck was going on with my Reynaud's!

The doctor put his finger on the pulse in my wrist and held my arm over my head. "Did anyone ever tell you you have thoracic outlet compression?" he asked.

"No, I don't."

Mom had nothing on me when it came to denial.

"It's a simple choice," he said. "Keep playing the drums and die. Stop playing and live."

Okay, it's not that I was really thinking this over, it's more that I was shocked to find out anything could possibly be wrong with me beyond the Reynaud's, which was familiar and workable, and on which I blamed absolutely everything that hurt or didn't work in my body since, let's remember, there was nothing else wrong with me.

Still, I hesitated long enough for Tom to bark, "What the fuck, Harris?! We're selling your drums and that's it!"

Which we did, to my AFM union rep, for a lot less than they were worth, but enough to make that month's rent.

So fine: now I knew what was wrong with me. Did TOC cause my horrible headache? No. What did cause it? Don't know. What should I do for this new congenital problem?

"Try not to use your right arm too much."

Wow. What great advice. It went right along with how to handle Reynaud's: "Try not to get too cold." So it was all just a question of not doing.

Hey, I could not do with the best of them.

We had to keep paying rent and buying milk, so Tom gigged for $35 here and $50 there—we never made that little on the road—

and I did more stupid temp jobs, at one of which I actually fell asleep and was told, believe it or not, to go home. While I tried to stay awake and Tom tried to revive his career as a solo pianist, he and I and our off-the-road road manager, Mike, wrote a book about playing the clubs.

Mike was a 6'9" scary-looking guy we met one day when I went up to him, baby in stroller, and said, "You look like someone who could move a refrigerator." He blinked at me, moved the refrigerator for us, and fell in love with our baby daughter all in one swell foop. One of the longer and more interesting interludes in our lives.

When it became clear I absolutely could not perform anymore, the three of us took to advising other, younger groups about the music business. This, naturally, let to the aforementioned book, which I wrote and they critiqued and took out my jokes.

Not knowing anything whatsoever about the book business, I sent the manuscript off to the five biggest publishers who put out books about the music industry. This was the late 1980s—long before the book business flipped on its ear, spun around three times, and spat over its left shoulder—so the two largest of them, Cherry Lane and Billboard Books, got into a fifteen-second bidding spat over our kicky little title that would enjoy its fifteen minutes of fame when Adam Curry plugged it on MTV.

We went with the top dollar offered by Watson-Guptil, owners of Billboard. That check, split three ways with our two shares lumped together, covered...just about nothing.

"Has anyone ever told you that writers don't make any money off the books they write?"

"Yes, they do," I insisted.

Sometime during his last stay in the hospital about a week before he died, my husband asked me, "Don't you ever get tired of being wrong?"

I said, "No, I'm pretty much used to it by now."

WHAT DIDN'T WORK, PART 1

Between 1985 and 1987, my body turned on me. There's no other way to look at it. I was going along, dealing with the tiredness, the headaches, the occasional vertigo, the general feeling of weakness that cropped up now and then, and the ever-present Reynaud's, on which I still pretty much blamed everything. If something else was wrong with me, well, I just handled that, too. Life goes on. I had a baby to support and a husband to bicker with.

And then I went blind. Totally. In the blink of one eye.

I freaked.

That's when I found out I had a "textbook" case of Reynaud's, because while waiting for a neurologist to show up in yet another emergency room, I started shivering and blanching. I'd been in and out of ERs a number of times by that point, always with the same result: "Have some naproxen. Diagnosis: probable M.S. (which I didn't believe)." We were at the Orange County Hospital this time, which was long ago taken over and immensely improved by UCI, but was, even then, a teaching institution. Instead of rushing in with extra blankets as Tom requested when I started shivering uncontrollably, every intern and resident in the place—and probably some woken from their off-time sleep—crowded into my tiny curtained enclosure to exclaim, "Look at her fingers!"

"Wow, feel her nose."

"Just like in the textbook."

"Can you take off your shoes so we can see if your feet are white?"

No, I couldn't. I was shaking too hard and my upper back had turned to brick, as it always did during a Reynaud's attack. God bless my lousy memory, I don't know how long it took for someone to show up and chase them all away or if that's even what happened at all. I'd like to think Tom did it, but I recall nada, zip, zilch after the textbook flurry.

The next day I saw a specialist who gave me another fun label, "optic neuritis," and told me that a) this was probably the onset or worsening of multiple sclerosis, and b) my days of wearing contact lenses were over.

Doctor…damn, his was an important name. I liked this one. I remember his lab room and his waiting room—unless that was some other guy's waiting room—but not his name or his face. Oh well, la-de-dah.

I think it was after my second or third visit that our always-on-its-last-spark-plug, non-gig-worthy car broke down. It was either a Pinto or a VW. Probably a Pinto. My vision had returned enough to drive (legally, albeit not safely) but not, apparently, enough to view anything with intelligence, because even though I already suspected (actually knew) I was pregnant, I pushed the car out of traffic and up the incline road to a safer, flatter spot.

By myself.

Later that evening, I was no longer pregnant.

I lost five babies in all. *Baruch Hashem* for Ilona.

In case you've never had a miscarriage, here's how it goes. First, you have sex. We did that, sporadically enough that Tom's sperm count was always high. During one episode of coitus or another, you get the sense that you just got pregnant. I always knew. I'm not unique: lots of women know. But I think I knew because by then I was so attuned to what was going on in my corporeal mass that I felt every minor tickle and wrinkle.

Buh Bye, MS.

One might say I was somewhat obsessed, but then One and I never got along well anyway, so One can just keep One's mouth shut.

You miss your period. I did that. You come up on the next, or miss it entirely. The part of your mind that knew you were pregnant says, "See? I told you so!" The part of your mind that insists no one can simply tell when they're pregnant says, "Shut up."

Then you start to bleed. Not like a normal period. It hurts more. And differently. A bad cramp comes along and you sit on the chamber pot and pass something that could simply be a clot. But as soon as it evacuates from your body, you burst into tears.

Miscarriage.

The last one I had was a fooler. Not only did I not think I was pregnant, I was pretty sure I had already started menopause. No period for almost four months at forty-eight seemed like peri-menopause to me. Then I got clobbered with the kind of contractions I remembered from having Lona, followed by an achingly painful start of my period, during which a long—I can't say finger-long, because my fingers are short and it was longer than them—very dense mass ripped out of my privates and into the waiting water. The pain backed off, the tears burst forth, and an hour later when they stopped, I knew.

Miscarriage.

Why didn't I go to a doctor for any of these episodes? you ask. Well, there's the rub. Tom was a musician; by then I was a ghostwriter. We lived off the grid of society, on the perimeter of all-that's-good-and-acceptable in the world. I fell between all medical-coverage cracks: too broke to sustain insurance, not broke enough to qualify for government help, although the state did once classify me as unemployable.

Not disabled, just unemployable. I had no idea what that meant. I don't think the guy at the welfare office to whom I showed the letter knew, either. What did it mean to the person who typed it up? Meaningless words meant to put me in my place? Or a helpful phrase that would pave the way to…what?

Not having access to AMA treatment was probably my saving grace, because it forced me to look elsewhere for help when my uterus voided another potential baby, my legs refused to propel me forward, my spine found better things to do than hold me up, my hands forgot the meaning of "grasp," the electricity running up and down my back could charge a car battery, or my sphincter went out for an unscheduled coffee break.

For the record, there is no other experience quite like stopping at a red light and realizing your bladder is emptying itself right then, right there, as you sit. No pain, no warning—in fact, no sensation at all in that one place of all places where you always want some kind of sensation, even if it's horrifically bad, which this wasn't. It was nothing. And I couldn't stop it. My mind screamed, "Noooooooooo!" and my nervous system said, "Huh? What? You talking to me?"

In the back of my head, I could hear the damn M.S. laughing.

"So, you think you can control me with all your vitamins and holistic crap? Well, take that!"

Lesson learned. From that time forth (I'd like to say it was the first and last time this happened. That's what I'd like to say. I really would), I never let my bladder be full or even half full, or semi, quasi, slightly containing anything. I emptied myself every sixty to ninety minutes, slipping away from wherever I was and back again with nothing but a head tilt or smile as comment.

This wasn't stoicism. This was war.

The last time I saw a doctor about my "probable M.S." was in some kind of clinic with a lot of corridors in which I got lost. The leaving part was the only good thing about the visit because when he said, "Reconcile yourself to a wheelchair," I said, "Fuck you!"— which would have been such a great exit line if it had been followed by my striding out of the room with my head held high.

Except, at the time, I was purposely not using a cane because, damn it, I wasn't going to use a cane (or two). So instead of striding, I stumbled, hit the wall, stumbled some more, and generally did a perfect imitation of someone who needed to reconcile herself to a wheelchair.

Buh Bye, MS.

I could recite the myriad hurdles my many-tentacled antagonist threw at me, but to what end? Take a look at any list of possible multiple sclerosis symptoms. At one point or another, I probably had all of them, although, of course, I don't remember. Each new incursion just got me angrier and angrier. Who the hell did this fucking dis-ease think it was?

A long, protracted war.

WHAT DIDN'T WORK, PART 2

While waiting for my full sight to return, which took about eighteen months in all, I saw a macro-biologist recommended by my friend Thelma. He told me that if my blood-test numbers were reversed, I'd have a perfect case of AIDS.

I hadn't a clue what AIDS had to do with me, but it shook me enough that I forgot the advice of one of my nursing-school teachers: "You need to mobilize anxiety in the patient to ensure compliance."

My anxiety was mobilized. I complied. He put me on a diet of various whole grains with familiar and exotic vegetables to be cooked no more than three minutes. No meat. No fruit. No sugar or chocolate. I, in my adorable innocence, thought, "Hey, a month or so of this and I'll get rid of those five pounds I want to lose, too."

However many months later I stopped (I want to say eight but I suspect I didn't make it that long—I certainly didn't make it very long without chocolate; what, are you kidding?), I was thirty-five pounds heavier and felt worse than ever before. I'd never weighed that much in my life. And while I'd previously struggled with monthly constipation as many women in my family did, my bowels had now ground to a complete stop.

Much, much later we figured out that my body doesn't process whole grains; it stores them in my joints where they can cause pain and stiffness. I take Whole Grain Cheerios as a personal affront. My corporeal mass doesn't like soy, either, but that didn't stop me from forcing tofu dinners on my family.

I deliberately didn't notice notice that Tom took his daughter "out for a ride" a lot more than usual during this period, with the two of them smelling of Naugle's burritos or Burger King fries on their return.

Macrobiotics was no good for any of us.

I went back to eating like a person, but I didn't lose any weight and I certainly didn't come back to where I'd been before I met Dr. InverseOfAIDS. That's the thing about multiple sclerosis: there's no going back. You might figure out how to stand your ground for a while, but you can never regain what you've lost.

Or so it wants you to believe, the lying, capricious little shit of an invasive maggot.

Next up: acupuncture and Eastern herbs. By now we'd moved out of the slums of Orange, where the Hillside Strangler hid out in the gravel pit behind our complex for a day or two. (Hovering police helicopters. Officers pacing the grounds with guns drawn. Every mother finding something for her kids to do inside, get in the house, right now, come inside, I mean it, now!)

We'd also moved out of the sweet Tustin apartment where Tom's brother-by-love slept on our couch Friday nights so he could watch *Pee Wee Herman's Playhouse* with his niece, my daughter, and then hurry to the Harlequin Theater to do a Saturday matinee and evening show before driving back to San Diego. The mother across the way made her son and daughter play together whether they wanted to or not because, she said, after she and her husband were gone, they would only be the only family each other had.

Wow. A revelation.

But after somebody cased The Van—it wasn't hard; everyone in the county knew that paint job—and burglarized it while we were on our once-a-month movie date, we moved back to Orange in a nice duplex where our six-month-old kitten could run down the long hallway from Lona's room to the front door, shoot up the screen to get a good push off, and then speed down the hall to make another turn-around on the bed. Good times.

Our biggest problem had to do with our landlord's contempt for renter's rights. His popping into our front or backyard whenever he felt like it seemed like a minor issue at the time.

I was taking a slew of vitamins and supplements, all expensive, none remembered, whose their benefits were negligible at best, detrimental at worst. The smell of Eastern herbs literally cleared the house whenever I cooked them up, and getting them down my gullet introduced me to the wonderful world of gag reflexes—but I drank/ate/swallowed it all, ever hopeful.

Well, mostly hopeful.

Not always hopeful.

I recall laying on the couch one afternoon—my normal position after 2:00 PM since my functioning hours were severely restricted but I kept working because, damn it! I Was Not Disabled!—when it occurred to me that I knew what our living-room ceiling looked like from every angle.

I was low enough at that point to intricately work out a foolproof suicide plan that (spoiler alert) never got enacted, but only because I was too fatigued to get up and do it. Nevertheless, I was sure the world, and certainly my family, would be better off without me as Public Burden #1.

Fatigued. Yes, I was using M.S. terminology by then. I hadn't been formally diagnosed and Mom had yet to pry open that locked vault in the back of her brain, but even an idiot could tell that everything I contended with regularly sounded amazingly just exactly like multiple sclerosis: imbalance, lack of grip, sporadically blurred vision, difficulty swallowing, slurred speech, a spine that scoffed at the evolutionary concept of humans walking in an upright position, and fatigue, fatigue, fatigue. Not a need to sleep; a need to go down. A need to stop.

A need to put my finger on whatever thought I was trying to put my finger on and an inability to do so.

Buh Bye, MS.

I was popping supplements as if they were helping. I was getting as much accomplished as possible in whatever time I had before my "switch went off," as my husband put it, and I was thereafter useless until the next morning. (I always felt better in the morning.) I was making healthy food and combining my victuals properly. I had a positive attitude, damn it, damn it, damn it. But I could do our taxes three times and come out with three different results, and I was slowly losing inches of territory every day.

Then, in March, 1994, I had an aortic spasm.

It felt like a heart attack. I was sure it was a heart attack. It started at the end of a long walk, which I took at least once a day to exercise since I no longer went to the gym (let's don't go there). This particular day, instead of my head clearing, my heart started racing halfway through my usual course, but I dismissed that. I was walking to calm my anger, so of course my heart would be racing.

By the time I got to the archway over our front path, I could barely breathe. I literally dropped to my knees, crawled inside, and dragged myself into the recliner. My breastbone was trying to shove through my backbone. The left side of my neck was about to burst, and the pain went both down my left arm and all the way south to the left side of my groin.

Tom came in and demanded to know what was going on. I couldn't talk to answer, but I forced myself to say "Remedy," because I also couldn't allow myself to pass out. I knew the moment I lost consciousness someone would call the paramedics, I'd be transported to an emergency unit, and I'd die. I knew that, absolutely, no question, even as I struggled to contain myself in my body, because a really big part of me wanted to leave so, so badly, right then; wasn't it time? The pain wasn't subsiding; it was just getting worse.

Tom fed me Rescue Remedy every fifteen minutes for the next two hours. I finished the bottle, dropperful by dropperful. The following day, I went to the doc-in-the-box around the corner where the M.D. on duty declared I'd had a moderately severe myocardial infarction, and hooked me up to an EKG machine to show me just how damaged my heart now was.

But it wasn't. There was no damage. I hadn't had an MI. And that really pissed him off.

My heart rate that day, maybe slightly fast, was perfectly normal and my heart murmur couldn't have caused what I'd described. He was furious—not at me, not really—but furious just the same. Imagine how I felt. I dragged around for over a month before feeling halfway human again.

The big news out of that fun adventure was that I had a heart murmur. He'd said it in passing, as if I already knew, which meant… what? Not a clue. Really, as I look back at all this, whenever I thought I had some semblance of being on top of things, it's distressing how clueless I was. It reminds me of the M.S. Society lunch Tom and I went to once where they handed out a chart that showed what doctors *used* to think M.S. was but "now we know" it to be something else. I couldn't help thinking that in a few years their happy conclusions could easily be just another line on the chart.

I went home from the doc-in-the-box and added my new label to the list: Reynaud's, Thoracic Outlet Syndrome, Probable Multiple Sclerosis, Heart Murmur.

"Wheat, Bera insisted. "Wheat is what's destroying your immune system. Wheat and meat."

So I became a vegetarian, one that didn't eat wheat of any kind. Two years. Didn't help. Gained weight.

That's right: I *gained weight* as a vegetarian.

I went vegan for eight months. It didn't help. I gained *more* weight and knew in the depths of my soul that God hated me. It was the only conceivable answer.

I did a naturopathic detox that took a lot of expensive ingredients and made a major mess in the kitchen. Didn't help.

I did a supplement-based detox. Didn't help. On the upside, it did cost a lot. Okay, not such an upside.

We got turned onto Evening Primrose Oil via a book, *Multiple Sclerosis,* I believe—catchy title, eh?—written by someone in England who was also battling M.S. and who had discovered that people with M.S. actually need red meat (thank you, thank you, Lord! *Ba-*

ruch Hashem). After the enormous build-up the author gave Evening Primrose Oil, our hopes were as high as an elephant's eye, but no, it only helped a little, not enough, and at the time, it was not all that readily available.

Hard to find and hardly worth it. What a combo!

I added a lot of shrimp to my diet to support my thyroid. It wasn't thyroid. I'd forgotten that. Tom had remembered, but the book said shellfish was good for me, the red meat of the sea. I never really followed that correlation, but I still eat shrimp when I can't get my hands on meat.

The meat actually needed to be steak. Hamburger was too processed to work. Chicken and pork, while more affordable, were just calories that filled me up but did nothing for my stamina or lucidity. Skirt steak was best because, at the time, it was cheap. I was high maintenance in the extreme.

By 2000, I was in very much not good shape. I seldom went to family parties or even to hear Tom perform anymore, because I could not tolerate the layers of sound, especially with the ringing in my ears providing the base. I'd had to use a wheelchair to get around the museums when we visited Chicago for Lona's sixteenth birthday, and had once flung myself out of the car—okay, wrenched myself awkwardly out of the car—in furious tears because Tom wanted me to either use an automatic cart to get around Costco, or wait for him to do the shopping.

I used a cane (or two) and sat down a lot—not easy in a store— just so I wouldn't have to use a wheelchair. Lona got one in the house for an art project and kept it around just in case. I refused to even sit in it. I couldn't drive at night at all, and I "let" my daughter chauffeur me around during the day. (I had been "letting" her drive me around since she was fourteen, maybe twelve, when we got her a hardship permit.) Fatigue hung on me like overgrown vines, holding me back, tripping me up, weighing me down. I went on eating binges to salve my depression and took cayenne pepper in capsules to keep the Reynaud's at bay. I figured I had another couple, maybe five years before the end.

I was formally diagnosed that the year with chronic multiple sclerosis—not remitting-relapsing; yeah, what a surprise—by Dr. Stanley VanderNoort of UCI, who saw me as a charity case after the Multiple Sclerosis Association of America (MSAA) paid for a diagnostic MRI. He talked with me at length because, he said, Reynaud's and multiple sclerosis is not really a good combination. I offered to drop one. He laughed. The point was, with the way my M.S. was progressing and the severity of my Reynaud's, anything he might prescribe for the one could negatively impact the other, and vice versa.

VanderNoort, whose name I could easily be misspelling, is the one who immediately recognized my non-myocardial infarction as an aortic spasm, and assured me that if I had gone to an emergency room, yes, they would have no doubt treated me for heart attack and yes, I indeed would have probably died. How fortunate I managed to stay conscious. I should work on that ability, and if it ever happens again, he cautioned, I should avoid going to an emergency room, because not only are M.S. and Reynaud's not really a good combination, the mitral valve prolapse (renamed from heart murmur) and thoracic outlet compression (TOC, re-acronym'd from TOS) didn't help matters.

The last thing he said to me was, "Keep taking that cayenne pepper."

So there I was, sitting in a rocking chair in the living room of our three-bedroom, one-family rented 1950s hand-built farm house, talking to my husband and daughter one fine September day in 2000, discussing something of some import, God alone knows what it was at this point, when my lungs stopped.

They just stopped.

No in-out, no deep breath, no air movement whatsoever—and, as with my earlier sphincter incidents, no manual control, either.

My brain screamed, "BREATHE!"

My lungs said, "Nope."

Buh Bye, MS.

A few eternal moments later, they started again, in-out, as if nothing had ever gone wrong, as if they'd never stopped, as if nothing had happened; what was I making such a fuss about?

Oh! I just remembered what we'd been talking about: funeral arrangements in the event of what seemed like my imminent death. And that was *before* my lungs went on hiatus.

I gave away my clients. I'd been teaching a rudimentary class onf how to be a ghostwriter for a few years against the possibility that sometime in the distant future I would need help. Obviously, I'd come to that time. This was it. My career was over.

I was ended.

WHAT DID WORK, PART 1

In early December 2000, financial circumstances, coupled with a man who actually uttered the words "Money is no object" and agreed to what was then the most outrageous fee I could imagine, forced me to take one last high-paying, even higher-stress ghostwriting gig. By January, I had stomach pains that acted like an ulcer. "Acted like," as in no, I didn't get tested or treated. I could not bear the thought of lugging around yet one more medical label, one more step toward the great beyond.

Bera, who had been recommending this protocol and that, and charting (I now find out) my stunning lack of progress throughout the years, had also been insisting I take noni juice for, oh, a long time. That winter, she worked out a deal with the South Pacific Trading Company for me to buy it at a greatly reduced cost so I would finally ("Please! Please! I'm begging you!") give this toxic-tasting 100% pure, expeller-pressed juice a try.

Starting sometime in early February, 2001, I drank three ounces of moni every morning. Bera wanted me to drink it twice a day, but while it tasted like Parmesan cheese to my landlady, to me it tasted like the bottom of a sewer. Not good-tasting stuff. I downed it from a glass in my left hand, followed immediately with an eight-ounce glass of water from my right.

Blech, blech, pftui, ew, blech!

Buh Bye, MS.

In July, 2001, my daughter and I drove Bera and Ron's 10-wheeler moving van from Orange, California to Bernalillo, New Mexico, which is just about three tumbleweeds past Albuquerque on the left.

In the heat.

With night vision.

And energy.

ENERGY.

Real, honest-to-God energy, the kind I hadn't had since...well, never. I'd never had so much energy, not at any previous point in my entire life.

When I came home and went back to work, I discovered that what used to take three months I could now accomplish in three or four weeks. Weeks!

Would the noni have been as effective if I hadn't readied my system with all those supposedly useless supplements and detoxes beforehand? If I hadn't done a liver cleanse three or four times a year? If I hadn't laid off grains (ALL grains) as much as possible and didn't chomp down broccoli like it was the latest blend of nectar and ambrosia?

Maybe, maybe not. How would I know? I can't even remember all the things I swallowed, rubbed in, and slurped up that didn't work. But the noni juice did. I felt better than I had in decades. Noni juice was a miracle!

But not a cure.

The cure—the two icing-on-the-cake elements that dissipated multiple sclerosis so entirely that it could not sustain itself in my carcass and had to slink away whimpering like the pathetic, slimy maggot it is—was a one-two punch from my wacky but loveable client in Mississippi and the zero-point field.

Remember the zero-point field? The one via which Tom and I were psychically connected?

Yeah, that one.

WHAT DID WORK, PART 2

I drank the undiluted noni juice straight, water chaser, for at least eighteen months. Part of my brain wants to say it was closer to two-and-a-half years. At that point, I switched to noni capsules, which were less expensive and certainly easier to swallow. Same effect, though. I felt good.

I still had to deal with some lingering problems, of course. My balance didn't balance. The stasis stayed. The headaches changed their visitation schedule at will. My night vision came and went, as if it was a poor relation. ("Fish and family stink after three days," my mother-in-law always reminded me. My night vision must have had the same mother-in-law.) And I took on a new label: optic migraines. Very pretty visually: interlocking triangles of color in a curve that start out tiny on the outside of the field of vision, and then grow as they flow ever so slowly to the other side. They're completely distracting, usually last some 20-25 minutes, and then fade away, to be immediately replaced by, of course, a brain-wracking headache.

"Don't worry," the ophthalmologist said. "It's usually a one-time occurrence."

I was not usually. Nothing in my body played out the way the books said it should. The migraines became part of my repertoire.

Buh Bye, MS.

Tom, Bera, and I tried to look at the creep that had invaded my systems from different angles and made some logical deductions. M.S. was akin to an electrical problem. My impulses weren't making it through my wires. Why?

Inflammation and spasm.

To reduce inflammation, I relied on arnica. I used both the homeopathic tablets (Hyland or Borion, didn't matter which) and the topical gel. I preferred Roberts Research Laboratories Arnica Gel; absorbs quickly, works well, and smells nice. If things got severe, I could take more tablets and reapply the gel every fifteen minutes. If that didn't work, I defaulted to left-over naproxen; I'd made a lot of ER visits over the years. But naproxen isn't good for my internal organs (I forget which one it affects. Liver? Kidneys? Gallbladder? One of those. Maybe the stomach. Whatever), so I stalled on taking it except in extreme instances.

My mother let me smear arnica gel on her leg after she had knee-replacement surgery. It always helped bring down the swelling, which relieved the pain. I gave her a tube of her own, and it only didn't help when she didn't use it. I have found this to be true across the board: if you don't rub it in (or dissolve it under your tongue, depending on which form you're using), it doesn't work at all. Not even a little. Doesn't sound reasonable, does it? But I've done this experiment over and over, and the result is always the same. Use it, it helps. Don't use it, it doesn't. Sometimes life is so amazing.

Bach Rescue Remedy took care of the spasms probably 97.86% of the time. Three dropperfuls under the tongue repeated as often as necessary, which was usually not more than two or three times per flare-up. In extreme, incorrigible episodes, I popped a left-over robaxin, a pharmaceutical anti-inflammatory. I'm sure both allopathic drugs were long past their expiration dates, but they still worked on those rare occasions when the arnica and Rescue Remedy didn't pull it off.

When I got too fatigued, my husband ran out and bought potato chips. Not the healthy baked or vegetable kind. The old-fashioned, greasy, salty kind. The salt-grease combination made me feel better, stronger, and less tired. Why?

Because. That's it. Because. Onacounta. Due to the fact. Whatever the reason, it worked. I didn't think I needed to know why.

Tom speculated that the greasy salt helped my electrical system, and he had a rational, remarkably plausible explanation for how and why it worked. It was a fine, inspirational discourse. I guess I should feel lucky that I remember the fact of it, if not the actual account.

By the way: yogurt, not so much. It was supposed to make me feel better and feed the healthy bacteria in my gut, but it just made me queasy. Go figure. Bera said my body was backwards: everything I did according to Hoyle didn't work. Everything that shouldn't help, did. Tom said some doctor once told me I was a drug reactor. I always took his word for it, because I don't remember that, either.

"Memory problems getting noticeably worse."

Were Tom here now, he'd roll his eyes, heave a massive sigh, and walk away, so just take that as given.

Between the noni, arnica, and Rescue Remedy to combat the M.S., and the cayenne capsules to keep the Reynaud's at bay, I did fairly well for a couple of years. I certainly handled my more debilitating symptoms better than most of the other people we know who had M.S. Our piano-player friend crawled into a bag of cocaine when he got his diagnosis and quickly ended up bedridden. The people I met at the support meetings were all resigned to daily injections and inevitable decline, and got together every week to keep each other's spirits up.

Gotta stay positive! Don't let yourself get depressed! If you do, remember to get an antidepressant from your doctor!

I never lasted long in those support groups; they made me too damn angry. What in the world were these people doing, giving up without a fight? Didn't they know multiple sclerosis was not just a physical adversary? It was a sonofabitch bloodsucking leech that had to be resisted and hammered against as if it were a Nazi cyanide shower! Why were they letting themselves be led into the death chamber like sheep? This was not God's will, damn it all to hell!

Sorry, I had to get that off my chest.

Buh Bye, MS.

With the new regimen, we pushed the interloper back to remitting/relapsing with just a few always-present exceptions: the visual distortions and limitations, the lack of balance, the tenuous sphincter compromise, and blah, blah, blah. BUT—if I lived carefully, which I mostly did (mostly), I'd get along for the rest of my life without any canes, wheelchairs, or allopathic interventions.

That's what I was aiming for; that's what I got.

In early 2003, a former client sent me a new client: wacky, wonderful Ron. Wacky, wonderful Ron lived on the other side of the country, had a great story to tell, and had been part owner of a supplement company that owned the patent on Superior Antioxidant Oral Chelation Formula. He claimed I simply *had* to try it. Besides a long list of nutrients, it had a proprietary blend of minerals and nutraceuticals (don't ya just love new made-up words?) that would change my life.

Okay...

But it was free and as Arthur Godfrey used to say, "For free, you take." So I took. When the first bottle showed up, I sent a copy of the label to Bera, who said, "Go ahead. It won't hurt you."

Oh, goody, because I just loved taking handfuls of supplements that wouldn't hurt me. But I'm diligent if nothing else, so I followed the recommended build-up program—one mornings and evenings for a week, then two twice a day, etc.—until I reached maintenance of three in the morning and two at night. It became part of my daily regimen, just another couple, three tablets in my cup of pills that, of course, included the cayenne and noni capsules, an Omega 3-6-9 gel cap to improve brain function, and an Aloelax capsule for...obvious reasons.

Ron kept sending me bottles of chelation, I so kept taking it. After a couple of years—yes, years—I noticed my night vision getting better. A few years later, I noticed I felt stronger—a strange thing to feel, I admit, but remember: I used to be a drummer. I knew what it felt like to be strong at least part of the day.

By the time Tom's mother died in May 2005, I felt pretty darn sturdy. Vigorous, even, and able to do something about it, too. Eighteen months later, I'd had the pedal to the metal so hard for so long that Tom and I were, for the first time in our marriage, completely out of debt.

It was an occasion, I tell you. A veritable triumph for a disabled ghostwriter who, although she made good money per annum, was married to a club musician, which negated most if not all fiscal gains tax season after tax season. For the first time since we'd walked up the steps of Chicago City Hall, thanks to having more vigor than I'd ever had before in life (Noni + Chelation = Energy[4]), the credit-card debts were gone, the financing debts were gone, and the IRS had Offer-and-Compromised out.

It didn't last, of course, but that wasn't anyone's fault. Sometimes shit happens. In October 2006, stuff that had nothing whatsoever to do with me or my squatter-infested body came along to strain our finances, our marriage, and our life in general.

It all ended as badly as humanly possible, but thanks to Tom's and my connection via the zero-point field, I finally shed the last vestiges of multiple sclerosis.

WHAT DID WORK, PART 3

It took me a long time to get to this part of the story. I may not have a good excuse for the delay, but I have a dandy explanation: I didn't want to write it.

When we last left our reluctant storyteller—that would be me—she had wrestled her intruder, a.k.a. multiple sclerosis, to a virtual standstill. The symptoms were chronic but no longer progressive, and nothing new had darkened the horizon for quite a while, health-wise.

Lest you think I did this all by myself, let me assure you I had more help than Houston has during a shuttle launch. My parents supported me emotionally, physically, and monetarily throughout the entire nasty affair. My daughter Lona gave up vast stretches of her childhood, youth, and young adulthood to drive for me, fetch for me, remember for me, do for me, worry for me, and sometimes even think for me. Bera researched, suggested, denounced, prodded, guided, and did everything but slap me upside the head with a two-by-four to help me. My client, Ron—bless his wacky, wonderful heart—kept sending those chelation tablets. My friends all deserve a presidential medal just for hanging with me all that time because I was never—trust me on this—stoic or silent. My mother-in-law, Doris, gave me the kind of support one might expect from a BFF without ever once making me feel I was too needy or intrusive.

And Tom...

And Tom.

Tom had a psychological break in October, 2006, almost exactly eighteen months after his mom died. It was as predictable and expected as Phoenix heat in July or wind down Michigan Avenue in the winter. Ever hear the musicians gag about the guy who knows he'll turn a corner in five years and someone will punch him in the nose? As much as I could have clocked Tom's crash with an egg timer, it was still a punch in the nose.

This was right in the middle of us acquiring the three young adults we took into our home (and hearts) and sent to community college. Tom balked at every single new person who came along until the point when he said, "Go get her!" about Tyger (a.k.a. Kathy) after Lona described Tyger's living conditions down in Texas; "Go get the cat!" about Nyxie (a.k.a. she doesn't like her real name so I won't use it) when he heard no one was actively caring for Taru the cat at her parents' house while she slept on our floor to avoid the 45-minute drive to and from work every day; and "Get your ass in here!" about Kata (a.k.a. Eric) when he was sleeping on our back porch because he'd gotten himself into trouble and had no place else to go and the weather had turned cold and rainy.

My husband was a very strict, hard-nosed guy with a soft, marshmallow center. As Skokie friend Scott wrote upon Tom's death, "His was a gentle soul with a bombastic spirit."

I have to believe our expanded family gave Tom something and someone else to worry about over the subsequent three and a half years of his life. I know he grew to love and cherish them, and to rely on every one of them, almost as much as he relied on Lona.

But, of course, he relied on me most of all.

Those years were very tough. He rallied now and then, but mostly he wanted to die. He had no plan. He wasn't actively suicidal. He was just done. The live-music business was going away. (Of course, it's beginning to revive again now—also predictable—in a haunting example of too little, too late.) He had finally finished his beloved History B.A. the previous semester, and was calf-deep in a master's program, but, "To what end?" we bantered endlessly. No one was going to give a fifty-year-old life-long freelance musician a straight job, no matter how many letters of recommendation he produced, or how many applications he painstakingly filled out. His position as a principal piano player at Knott's Berry Farm had become bone-achingly dreary, and his need for constant connection with me drainingly obsessive.

So we talked, which is to say, he talked, I listened. Ironically (or not), I had written a song for him called "I'll Still Listen" back at the beginning of our marriage. (He'd written one for me called "Just For Laughs," an unwitting foreshadowing of our lives together.)

He despaired. I encouraged. He grew nasty as he got more despondent. I grew angry and bitter as I got more impatient.

And the M.S. gave way, just a little bit.

Huh?

We both put on weight, which gave him more cause to lose hope. I hated the way I looked, but could not help noting that for all my extra poundage, I physically felt better.

Was my miserable parasite morphing from my physique and invading his psyche?

In November, 2009, I took him to Western Medical Center emergency room—talk about your turnabouts. Doubled over in pain, he "knew" he had another kidney stone, that's how bad it hurt, and demanded Toridol, if that's the right spelling, for the pain. The damn ER doctor ignored his belligerent request and instead ran some tests.

It wasn't a kidney stone. It was pancreatis. Very painful. He spent three days in the hospital, hallucinating from continual doses of heavy pain medications and telling me to "Get the hell out of here."

I got the hell out.

I also jumped through a couple dozen hoops to get him on MSI, a county medical plan, so he could continue to get medical attention when he came home from the hospital. We weren't all that bad off financially, but no insurance company in its right corporate mind would ever consider thinking about possibly covering either one of us.

Instead of going to the clinic where I'd so painstakingly arranged for him to be seen, he continued to look for a straight job during the day and go out nights to break into the dueling-piano world. He was a natural. He had friends who would help him, hands that worked no matter what, and a stage charisma that made audiences smile.

But he was tired.

Tired was something I understood. My tiredness—not fatigue at this point, just tiredness—came from ghosting for my clients, creating the final edition of the definitive textbook on ghostwriting, teaching my expanded training program, handling the house, dealing with the kids and their school issues, and providing Tom almost nonstop psychological support. We tried going to a few actual therapists, but they did not give him what he wanted or needed, which became ever-obviously more and more of me.

I didn't voice it at the time, but in retrospect, the more of my time and energy he demanded, the less the M.S. did.

Huh.

On April 14, Tom turned fifty-eight playing what would be his last gig ever at the Villa Nova in Newport Beach. We'd sent word out that he was subbing that night, and friends and fellow musicians filled the room. The kids and I left after a few hours; I had to work in the morning and they had classes.

Everyone understood that Tom's pancreatitis was wearing him out.

The next day, I took him to the emergency room for pain. They sent him home with a few heavy-duty prescriptions. We didn't have time to fill them, though, because the day after that, he returned to Western Med via ambulance, spitting up blood.

I'm going to cut to the chase here because these memories, which sadistically remain intact, are too raw. Between April 16 and May 29, 2010, we went in and out of three different hospitals as one doctor after another got exasperated with Tom's calls for pain medication. He received first one, then six, then another six units of blood for what started as a bleeding, then segued into an obstructive, duodenal ulcer. His pain-med demands alienated every nurse and hospitalist who interacted with him, to the point that one gastroenterologist called me in the middle of a Saturday, and said he didn't want to have anything to do with my husband anymore. As soon as he was done running tests and discharged Tom, he was through. Good luck to you, lady.

On May 29, after that same gastroenterologist received the results of those tests, he recanted and sent Tom to UCI for an outpatient procedure to open his duodenal passage so the man could eat again. Forty-five minutes into the expected two-hour operation, I was called into the recovery area.

"I couldn't get the tube past his duodenum. He has Stage 4 cancer. It's already metastasized to his liver. He has six to twelve months. There's nothing we can do. You can leave whenever you're ready. I'm sorry."

Life changed.

I'm not going to go through that next month step-by-step. Use your imagination. Or don't. Wish my intermittent amnesia would kick in for some this, but it won't. Long story short: we made up for everything either of us had ever done or said to or about each other. We re-pledged our love. He proposed once more (for the umpteenth time). I accepted once more (for the umpteenth time). We played cards. I slept in the room every night and left to get coffee a lot so I didn't cry in front of him because it made him feel helpless. He promised to get well and take dance lessons with me and go on a cruise.

We both knew he was lying.

"If I can't eat," he had said as I wheeled him down the path from the UCI GI Outpatient Surgery Clinic, "I'll be dead in a month."

And so he was.

He died exactly one month later, June 28 at 10:35 AM. I was, by then, down to a single functioning brain cell. I did what I had to do, with enormous above-and-beyond help from my parents, my kids, my brother and sister-in-law, Tom's brother-by-love Leon, and my beloved rabbi, Bernie King, who died of his own liver disease six months later, *alev ha sholem*.

The M.S. did not make a single peep. Not the slightest whimper. Sure, I slept a lot, but that was grief. My hair fell out—textbook grief. I was beyond bereft. This man had been in my life for forty-two years.

Hmmm. Multiple sclerosis had been in my life for...forty-two years.

The sun kept coming up every single day. Tom stayed dead long after the joke stopped being funny. He'd sent me a song through Bera the day he died. I remember the fact and the feel of it, nothing more. I had a few stasis incidents that were utterly vanquished by absent-mindedly taking Rescue Remedy. I pushed on, worked through, cried myself to sleep, watched funny movies and endless repeats of *Whose Line Is It, Anyway?*

Tom had told me that after he died, I'd grieve for a little while, then find myself a man who'd treat me better than he ever did. I took no solace in the fact that, for once, he was incontrovertibly wrong.

By November of that year, I'd come to the end of my emotional rope and took off with Lona in the new, reliable vehicle I bought to replace The Van that, yeah, Tom had still been driving. We were only going to be gone for a day or two, so, throwing caution to the wind and not really caring one way or the other anyway, I took no supplements of any sort with me.

We were gone for six days. I was fine until my body reminded me that M.S. or no M.S., I was still a girl with a four-generation digestive dysfunction. Otherwise—no ill effects.

In January, I got sick as a dog with the flu. The flu?!

Understand: for decades, I never got sick. No cold, no flu. No bug could get very far in my body, which was in active search-and-destroy mode, killing off my nerve connectors and brain cells and—*wait, what's that? Something new? Kill it!*—whatever else had the audacity to penetrate my system. Now, I was on my back, coughing, wheezing, hacking, sneezing, whimpering sick for well over a week.

Buh Bye, MS.

Ha! The multiple sclerosis was laying down on the job.

It took me another few months of paying close attention to accept as reality that yeah, the enemy had been vanquished. Banished. Expelled, ejected, cast out.

It had ceased to exist.

Just like my never-to-be-recaptured memory lapses, it was gone, gone, gone.

Did Tom take it with him? Did my physical dreck leech into him and die along with his poor, cancer-ridden body? Did his soul, knowing he was about to shed his corporeal mass, suck it from mine?

Uh. Yeah.

WHAT DID WORK, FINALE

Eradicating M.S. was a process. Not a fast one, but one with permanent results. Looking back at the mutiny, I can grab onto a lot of what I did, although, obviously, not all of it. Tom took those exact recollections with him. But for those who are as stubborn and bitchy as I am and cannot conceive of surrendering their sword no matter how much territory they've lost, here's the rundown as best I can remember.

Again, a proviso: the following are not independent steps taken one at a time. I merely grouped them for explication.

First, I detoxed. A lot. Got off wheat and, in fact, ALL grains for a full eighteen months, twice. I did liver detoxes, colon detoxes, gallbladder detoxes, kidney and bladder detoxes. I cooked with coconut oil to help clear the plaque from my arteries. I took cayenne to strengthen my vascular system. I write all this in the past tense, but I still eat minimal wheat, no whole grains, and minimal sugar, including fruit.

I cook with coconut oil, still take cayenne capsules twice daily, and make sure my digestive track empties fully and easily every day without fail. "Death begins in the colon." Don't remember who said that, but I believe they're right.

Second, I built up. Lots of carrot juice: so much that the palms of my hands actually turned orange. Lots of broccoli and spinach.

69

Also lots of beets, but that's mostly because I love fresh-cooked, not-from-a-can beets, which I eat for breakfast with a dollop of sour cream.

Third, I avoided chemicals in food; yeah, I read labels. No, I don't love to cook and I never went strictly organic, but I gave up packaged foods and canned foods and frozen foods and other food-like substances. For the most part. I probably stayed good eighty-five to ninety percent of the time. When I fell off the wagon, I got right back on as soon as I could.

Fourth, I ate/eat meat. My two years as a vegetarian and eight months as a vegan were enormous mistakes. People battling M.S. need cow. I never worried about fat or cholesterol, never ate low-fat anything. I countered the cholesterol nonsense with the detoxes and the coconut oil and the cayenne.

Lots of health-oriented people advocate going non-dairy to reduce fat intake and avoid lactose problems. I go very dairy. My body craves cow. Sorry, but the Talmud says health comes first, and my health depends on beef. So I took bovine colostrum and made sure I had steak, not hamburger, a couple times a week. In fact, Tom insisted I leave him alone in the hospital on Sundays to go eat steak and eggs. Chicken and pork never helped. Shrimp did, some-what. Catfish didn't. Neither did cod, but that's okay because while I love fish and chips, my body doesn't appreciate the breading. For me—and maybe only me, I wouldn't know—grains equal pain and soy makes me sore. Protein, protein, protein (from beef) gave me strength. The powders and drinks and what-have-you were useless.

Fifth, I refused purposely, fervently, and with malice of fore-thought to think of myself as fragile. Ever. Don't go there: it's a trap, I promise you. I never accepted my condition as permanent. Never. I never said, thought, or even entertained, "Why me?" Never let my-self slide into victimhood. Never, never, never. I never stopped work-ing, even when I could only work for two or three hours a day—not at a time, *a day*. I learned to plant my feet so I was steadier. I learned to lean so I didn't feel like I had to fall. I learned to give my body what it needed at the moment, always reminding it that this condi-tion was not going to stand. I was coming back, somehow, someday, count on it. I learned to let other people's problems be theirs, not mine, which reduced a tremendous amount of external and unnecessary stress. I learned to release the anger and pain I harbored from my childhood, from my family, from my clients, from my circumstances. This part was sinisterly tough to accept at first, but was an absolute godsend afterwards. I learned to forgive, release, and move on.

And never look back—which, admittedly, is pretty easy when you don't really remember, anyway. I made a virtue out of necessity.

Six, the noni juice. *It single-juicidly changed my life.* I don't know that it would have been so effective if I hadn't set my body up for it, but I know for certain and for sure that noni truncated the disability my unworthy opponent kept trying to inflict on me. With noni, I could work full days. I could tolerate hot weather. My Reynaud's problems diminished. My night vision improved. My M.S. symptoms became manageable. For me, noni was a miracle.

Seventh, after years of all the above, I started that oral chelation. It took probably a year and a half to really make a difference, although I began feeling stronger about three or four months into the regimen. My night vision not only came back, my normal vision improved so much I no longer needed trifocals or even bifocals. My balance improved. The bodily functions I had to constantly monitor regulated. The combination of all of the above pushed the M.S. back so far, I barely acknowledged it as I went about my daily life.

Finally, I released it. Immediately after his death, while I was still actively communicating with Tom psychically, I told him, "I was diagnosed with this damn thing the year we met. If you have to leave to leave me, take it with you."

One day, a few weeks after my terrible bout of flu, I realized I wasn't watching my bladder. My vision was fine. I hadn't had a single optic migraine the previous summer. My balance was steady. I could hold a cup or a glass or a plate and not be concerned about dropping it. I felt everything in my body, everywhere: no dead areas, no numbness. No stasis across my back. No problem with heat whatsoever.

I felt it gone.

Buh Bye, MS.

I still feel it not here.

Sounds crazy, doesn't it? But I don't have multiple sclerosis anymore. The Reynaud's is utterly under control. My skin is clear, my eyes have no more discolorations (I'd gotten into iridology along the way; doesn't everyone?) my tongue is pink and rounded and full (shades of Chinese medicine), not flat. I have energy. I sleep well no matter what the weather. I can take deep breaths without resistance. My hair has grown back. My nails are hard as…well, nails.

Have I cured everything?

Nah.

The thoracic outlet compression that took away my career as a professional drummer remains, as does the mitral valve prolapse and slight scoliosis that, oh yeah, I forgot to mention (because I ignore it). None of that structural stuff affects me so long as I don't try to pretend I can now go out and be the athlete I never was. The memory problems remain, although sometimes I think they're getting better. My kids say they're getting worse. My husband knew how to work around my lack of recall, but it tends to drive my grown children nuts.

Bless it and release it, I tell them.

They roll their eyes.

EPILOGUE

It has been about two years since I wrote the last chapter, a good point at which to look back and see how things are progressing.

It's all good.

I now wear single-vision, long-distance glasses, because my eyesight has improved to the point that I see close things best with no correction at all.

My hair continues to grow in thicker and fuller.

My body is releasing the extra weight. I'm down from a size twenty-two pants jeans to a size sixteen, and they're getting too big.

I can do moderate exercise without it kicking back on the rest of my day.

No stasis. No sphincter lapses. No lung interruptions. Steady hands. Full-day functioning. Good nightly sleep.

And balance! I have balance. I do light yoga every day to improve my stability and instead of laughing at me, my body accepts it. So cool!

The M.S. remains eradicated, banished, vanquished.

(*I win, I win, nya nah na nah na.*)

APPENDIX: SUPPLEMENTS & FOOD

Antioxidant Oral Chelation

The brand I use is not available on the open market, but the Internet is full of other possibilities. Check with your naturopath or holistic doctor if you want advice on which to try. Chelation pulls the heavy metals and ammonia out of individual cells and from behind your eyes. No one has ever asked my opinion, but I truly believe that the upsurge in auto-immune problems has a lot to do with heavy-metal poisoning. This isn't something we can avoid in today's world of cars and trains and fertilizers and antiperspirants and advanced dentistry and microwaves and cell phones and all the other products and gizmos with which we live and on which we rely in our technologically advanced, civilized society. Taking an anthropological perspective, I can't help but see a correlation.

Cayenne

One capsule twice a day. More if I get cold. I use hot sauce on my eggs and in my cooking. The heat keeps my blood vessels open, my brain cells snapping, and my digestive track strong.

Omega 3-6-9.

'Cause. We all need it. I'm not that young anymore, who is? I can always use the brain boost and the oil to keep things flowing and flush of my various bodily systems. Speaking of which...

Aloelax and Cascara Sagrada

I know, I know: if I take these regularly, my body will become dependent on them. Well, if I don't, my body reverts to that four-generation digestive dysfunction I've alluded to altogether too many times. Do I have to spell it out? I don't mind being dependent on something that works. The way I figure it, I'm dependent on food, water, and air, too. Death ain't gonna begin in my colon, bucko. Give it up for addiction to effective evacuation!

Noni

I still take two capsules every morning. Do I still need it? Maybe, maybe not. Do I want to take the chance of stopping? As Tom would say, "What the fuck, Harris?!" Seriously.

Biotin and Silica

For healthy hair and nails. Lost 'em first with the M.S., again when Tom died. I like healthy hair and nails. Sue me; I'm a girl. My finger and toenails used to just tear off. Now they have to be cut because they're nail hard.

Milk Thistle, aka Silymarin

I go through a bottle of mild Silymarin three or four times a year to detox and support my liver, where all the junk from the environment and what I eat and drink ends up. I can't change the world outside, but I can make sure my innards stay clean and healthy.

Wheat

I fall off the wagon now and then, but in general I avoid it, especially whole-grain wheat. I'm not gluten intolerant, but wheat it hurts my knees and makes me retain water. Why? To steal from Professor Irwin Corey, the World's Greatest Authority, that's really two questions. Number one: "Why?" Why is a question that has plagued mankind since the beginning of time, and I'm certainly not going to try to answer it here and now. And number two: "Does wheat h my knees hurt and make me retain water?"

Yes.

Buh Bye, MS.

Soy

Soy is on my never-even-look-at-again list. I think I overdid it during all those "try this, try that" years. Now it goes right to the bottom of my spine and irritates my sciatica nerve. I know, I know, that doesn't make sense. But I've matched the reaction to the ingestion enough.

No soy. No miso. No tofu. No edamame.

My body, my choice.

Your body. Your choice.

Claudia Suzanne is a professional ghostwriter with nearly 120 invisible non-fiction and fiction credits. She lives in Orange County, California with myriad human and nonhuman folk and a computer that won't keep up with her.